T0292627

Urodynamics, Neurourology and Pelvic Floor Dysfunctions

The aim of the book series is to highlight new knowledge on physiopathology, diagnosis and treatment in the fields of pelvic floor dysfunctions, incontinence and neurourology for specialists (urologists, gynecologists, neurologists, pediatricians, physiatrists), nurses, physiotherapists and institutions such as universities and hospitals.

More information about this series at http://www.springer.com/series/13503

Antonio Carbone • Giovanni Palleschi
Antonio Luigi Pastore • Aurel Messas
Editors

Functional Urologic Surgery in Neurogenic and Oncologic Diseases

Role of Advanced Minimally Invasive Surgery

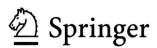

Editors
Antonio Carbone
Department of Medico-Surgical Sciences
and Biotechnologies
Sapienza University of Rome
Rome
Italy

Antonio Luigi Pastore
Department of Medico-Surgical Sciences
and Biotechnologies
Sapienza University of Rome
Rome
Italy

Giovanni Palleschi
Department of Medico-Surgical Sciences
and Biotechnologies
Sapienza University of Rome
Rome
Italy

Aurel Messas
Urologic Surgery
Max Fourestier Hospital
Nanterre
France

Urodynamics, Neurourology and Pelvic Floor Dysfunctions
ISBN 978-3-319-29189-5   ISBN 978-3-319-29191-8   (eBook)
DOI 10.1007/978-3-319-29191-8

Library of Congress Control Number: 2016940505

Printed on acid-free paper

This Springer imprint is published by Springer Nature
The registered company is Springer International Publishing AG Switzerland

"To our beloved lifelong companions and children, whose love, patience and constant support make every of our efforts a success"

Foreword

Functional surgery in oncologic and neuro-urological patients is one of the hardest tasks for urologists. The search for the ideal bladder replacement began as early as 1855 when Tuffier reported his experience with ureterosigmoidostomy. The use of isolated bowel segments started to be investigated in the 1950s. In the following decades, detubularization and reconfiguration optimized functional results in terms of low-pressure reservoir with good neo-bladder capacity. Open surgery is routinely adopted. In this book, authors report advanced minimally invasive surgical options using laparoscopy or robotics. Such new approaches have been shown efficacy with low risk of adverse events in the short and medium follow-up. These promising outcomes should be confirmed in the long term and possibly improved by means of further technological innovations and surgical experience.

Despite the amelioration of surgical techniques, stress urinary incontinence (SUI) is still a prevalent complication after radical prostatectomy or radical hysterectomy. This issue is taken into account by authors reporting mini-invasive solutions in both genders.

An overview of neurogenic dysfunctions and their specific treatment also in complicated clinical patterns such as the presence of pelvic floor pain and concomitant anatomical bladder outlet obstruction in chronic or progressive neurological disease is described in detail.

Bladder augmentation is the last option in the management of neurological patients with high risk of upper urinary tract deterioration. In neurological population, the primary aim is to achieve a low-filling-pressure high-capacity reservoir, as the voiding phase is obtained by self-intermittent catheterization. Entero-cystoplasty remains the gold standard despite being associated with multiple complications, such as metabolic disorders, calculus formation, mucus production, enteric fistulas, and potential for secondary malignancy. Clearly, this is an area of unmet needs and search for novel solutions.

Editors and authors are to be commended for their efforts to outline contemporary reconstructive functional urologic surgery.

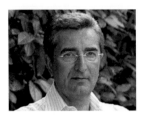

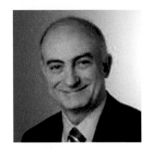

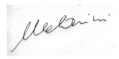

Marco Carini
Chief. of Urology
Unit – Oncology Department,
University of Florence,
Florence, Italy

Walter Artibani
Chief. Urology Unit,
University of Verona
Verona, Italy

Preface

This second book of the Italian Urodynamic Society (SIUD) addresses functional aspects of the lower urinary tract. In particular, this manuscript presents preventive measures in oncological patients who have undergone demolitive surgery with the use of new robotic and/or laparoscopic technology, as well as new minimally invasive techniques for reconstruction or functional recovery. Interestingly, for some aspects, the approach for recovering micturition control is similar in oncological and neurological patients as reported in the second part of the book. On behalf of SIUD, we believe to have provided a precious contribution, thanks to the editors and all authors who are internationally known as experts on this field, to interested readers who want to understand more functional urological surgery and who want to get ideas for implementing their knowledge about current or developing minimally invasive surgical procedures in functional urology. In closing, special thanks go to all coauthors who contributed to the fulfillment of this project.

I hope you will enjoy reading.

Florence, Italy   Giulio Del Popolo

Contents

Contributors

Youness Ahallal Department of Urology, Clinique de l'Alma, Paris, France

Samer Fathi Al-Rawashdah Urology Unit, Department of Special Surgery, Faculty of Medicine, Mutah University, Karak, Jordan

Yazan Al Salhi Urology Unit, Department of Medico-Surgical Sciences and Biotechnologies, Sapienza University of Rome, Latina, Italy

Matteo Bonifazi Department of Urology, Careggi University Hospital, Florence, Italy

Antonio Carbone Urology Unit, Department of Medico-Surgical Sciences and Biotechnologies, Sapienza University of Rome, Polo Pontino, Latina, Italy

Guido Carpino Department of Movement, Human and Health Sciences, University of Rome "Foro Italico", Rome, Italy

Davide Cavaliere Surgery and Advanced Oncologic Therapies Unit, Morgagni-Pierantoni Hospital, AUSL Romagna, Forlì, Italy

Giuseppe Cavallaro Department of Medico-Surgical Sciences and Biotechnologies, Sapienza University, Rome, Italy

Flaminia Coluzzi Department of Medico-Surgical Sciences and Biotechnologies, Unit of Anaesthesia, Intensive Care and Pain Medicine, Sapienza University of Rome, Rome, Italy

Simone Crivellaro Urology Department, University of Illinois at Chicago, Chicago, IL, USA

Giulio Del Popolo Neurourology Unit, Careggi University Hospital, Florence, Italy

Ryan W. Dobbs Urology Resident, PGY 2nd, University of Illinois at Chicago, Chicago, IL, USA

Enrico Finazzi Agrò Department of Experimental Medicine and Surgery, Tor Vergata University of Rome, Rome, Italy

Jacopo Frizzi Department of Urology, Careggi University Hospital, Florence, Italy

Andrea Fuschi Urology Unit, Department of Medico-Surgical Sciences and Biotechnologies, Sapienza University of Rome, Polo Pontino, Latina, Italy

Michele Gallucci Department of Urology, "Regina Elena" National Cancer Institute, Rome, Italy

Inderbir Gill Catherine and Joseph Aresty Department of Urology, USC Institute of Urology, Keck School of Medicine, University of Southern California, Los Angeles, CA, USA

Cristian Gozzi Urology Department, University of Pisa – Italy, Pisa, Italy

Alessandra Graziottin Center of Gynecology and Medical Sexology Hospital San Raffaele Resnati, Milan, Italy

Foundation for the Cure and Care of Pain in Women – NPO, Milan, Italy

David T. Greenwald Urology Resident, PGY 2nd, University of Illinois at Chicago, Chicago, IL, USA

Fabio Landoni Gynecology Department IEO, European Institute of Oncology, Milan, Italy

Monika Lukasiewicz IInd Department of Obstetrics and Gynecology, University of Warsaw, Warsaw, Poland

Medical Center for Postgraduate Education, Belanski Hospital, Warsaw, Poland

Vincenzo Li Marzi Department of Urology, Careggi University Hospital, Florence, Italy

Aurel Messas Urologic Surgery, Max Fourestier Hospital, Nanterre, France

Bart Morlion The Leuven Centre for Algology, University Hospitals Leuven, University of Leuven, Leuven, Belgique

Medical Faculty KU Leuven, Leuven, Belgique

Giovanni Mosiello Pediatric Urology, Bambino Gesù Hospital, Rome, Italy

Thomas J. Pallaria Department of Anesthesiology, Newark Beth Israel Medical Center – Rutgers University School of Medline, New Brunswick, NJ, USA

Giovanni Palleschi Urology Unit, Department of Medico-Surgical Sciences and Biotechnologies, Sapienza University of Rome, Latina, Italy

Antonio Luigi Pastore Department of Medico-Surgical Sciences
and Biotechnologies, Urology Unit, Sapienza University of Rome,
Latina, LT, Italy

Joseph Pergolizzi, MD Temple University School of Medicine,
Philadelphia, PA, USA

Johns Hopkins University School of Medicine, Baltimore, MD, USA

Vincenzo Petrozza Department of Medico-Surgical Sciences
and Biotechnologies, Sapienza University of Rome, Latina, Italy

Stefano Scabini Oncologic Surgery Unit, IRCCS San Martino Institute,
Genoa, Italy

Giuseppe Simone Department of Urology, "Regina Elena" National
Cancer Institute, Rome, Italy

Marco Soligo Obstetrics and Gynecology Department, Hospital Vittore
Buzzi, ICP, Milan, Italy

Anand Thakur Department of Anesthesiology, Wayne State University,
Detroit, MI, USA

Vanna Zanagnolo Gynecology Department IEO, European Institute
Oncology, Milan, Italy

Part I

Functional Urologic Surgery in Oncologic Patients

Functional Anatomy of Pelvic Organs

1

Guido Carpino, Vincenzo Petrozza,
and Samer Fathi Al-Rawashdah

1.1 Pelvic Cavity

The abdominopelvic cavity consists of the circular true (lesser) pelvis, wherein the urogenital organs lie, and the false (greater) pelvis which corresponds to the iliac fossae and is largely in contact with intraperitoneal contents.

The limit between true and false pelvis is represented by the pelvic inlet, a plane passing through the promontory of the sacrum, the arcuate line on the ilium, the iliopectineal line, and the posterior surface of the pubic crest [1].

The walls of the true pelvic cavity consist of sacrum and bony pelvis, ligaments interconnecting these bones, and the muscles lining their inner surfaces. Inferiorly, the pelvic outlet of the true pelvis is closed by the pelvic diaphragm (floor) which is a muscular partition formed by the levator ani and coccygei muscles. The lateral walls of the true pelvis are composed of the bony pelvis and the obturator internus and piriformis muscles.

The anterior and posterior iliac spines, the iliac crests, the pubic tubercles, and the ischial tuberosities are palpable landmarks that orient the pelvic surgeon [2].

G. Carpino
Department of Movement, Human and Health Sciences, University of Rome "Foro Italico", Rome, Italy

V. Petrozza
Department of Medico-Surgical Sciences and Biotechnologies, Sapienza University of Rome, Latina, Italy

S.F. Al-Rawashdah (✉)
Urology Unit, Department of Special Surgery, Faculty of Medicine, Mutah University, Karak, Jordan
e-mail: Samer.Rawashdah@gmail.com

© Springer International Publishing Switzerland 2016
A. Carbone et al. (eds.), *Functional Urologic Surgery in Neurogenic and Oncologic Diseases*, Urodynamics, Neurourology and Pelvic Floor Dysfunctions, DOI 10.1007/978-3-319-29191-8_1

1.2   Pelvic Muscles

The pelvic muscles form two groups: the first group is represented by piriformis and obturator internus which are also considered lower limb muscles and form the lateral wall of true pelvis; the second group is represented by levator ani and coccygeus which form the pelvic diaphragm and outline the lower limit of the true pelvis.

Piriformis forms part of the posterolateral wall of the true pelvis [1]: proximally, it is attached to the anterior surface of the sacrum, then passes out of the pelvis through the greater sciatic foramen, and attaches to the greater trochanter of the femur. The anterior surface of piriformis is related, inside the pelvis, to the rectum and to the sacral plexus of nerves and branches of the internal iliac vessels, while the posterior surface lies against the sacrum. *Obturator internus* forms part of the anterolateral wall of the true pelvis [1]. It is attached to the structures surrounding the obturator foramen and to the medial part of the pelvic surface of the obturator membrane; it leaves the pelvis through the lesser sciatic foramen and attaches to the trochanteric fossa of the femur. Ischiococcygeus (or coccygeus) represents the most posterosuperior portion of pelvic floor and arises as a triangular musculotendinous sheet with its base attached to the lateral margins of the coccyx and sacrum and its apex to the ischial spine and sacrospinous ligament. *Levator ani* forms a large portion of the pelvic floor and is attached to the internal surface of the true pelvis. The muscle is subdivided into iliococcygeus, pubococcygeus, and puborectalis. Levator ani arises from each pelvic sidewall along the tendinous arch of levator ani (the condensation of the fascia of the obturator internus). *Iliococcygeus* forms the lateral portion of the levator ani attached to the inner surface of the ischial spine and to the tendinous arch of levator ani while, medially, it is attached to the lateral margins of the coccyx and to the anococcygeal ligament. *Pubococcygeus* represents the medial portion of the levator ani and is attached to the back of the body of the pubis and passes back almost horizontally. The most medial fibers run directly lateral to the urethra and its sphincter as it passes through the pelvic floor; here the muscle is named the puboperinealis, although due to its close relationship to the upper half of the urethra in both sexes it is often referred to as pubourethralis. The muscle fibers from both sides form part of the urethral sphincter complex together with the intrinsic striated and smooth musculature of the urethra where fibers intersect across the midline directly behind the urethra. Then, the medial fibers run posteriorly and reach the anorectal junction and the deep part of the external anal sphincter, thus forming the puborectalis muscle. Posterior to the rectum, the fiber of the pubococcygeus crosses the midline forming a fibrous raphe, the anococcygeal ligament, which is attached to the coccyx.

1.3   Pelvic Fascias

The pelvic fascia is divided into the parietal pelvic fascia, which forms the coverings of the pelvic muscles, and the visceral pelvic fascia, which forms the coverings of the pelvic viscera and their vessels and nerves [1].

Parietal pelvic (endopelvic) fascia consists of the obturator fascia, the piriformis fascia, the levator ani fascia (superior fascia of pelvic diaphragm), and the presacral fascia. The *obturator fascia* is connected above to the posterior part of the arcuate line of the ilium and is continuous with iliac fascia. Anterior to this, as it follows the line of origin of obturator internus, it is gradually separated from the attachment of the iliac fascia and a portion of the periosteum of the ilium and pubis spans between them. It arches below the obturator vessels and nerve, investing the obturator canal, and is attached anteriorly to the back of the pubis. Behind the obturator canal, the fascia is markedly aponeurotic and gives a firm attachment to levator ani, called the tendinous arch of levator ani. *Piriformis fascia* fuses with the periosteum on the front of the sacrum at the margins of the anterior sacral foramina where it enchases the sacral anterior primary rami. *Levator ani fascia (superior and inferior fascia of pelvic diaphragm)* covers both the surfaces of the pelvic diaphragm. On the lower surface, the thin inferior fascia is continuous with the obturator fascia laterally below the tendinous arch of levator ani. It covers medially the wall of the ischioanal fossa and extends below to give fasciae on the urethral sphincter and external anal sphincter. On the upper surface, it is attached anteriorly to the back of the body of the pubis and extends laterally across the superior ramus of the pubis, blending with the obturator fascia and continuing to the spine of the ischium. *Presacral fascia* forms a hammock-like structure behind the posterior portion of the rectal fascia and extends laterally to the origin of the piriformis and levator ani fasciae. Inferiorly, it reaches the anorectal junction, fusing with the posterior aspect of the rectal fascia and the anococcygeal ligament at the anorectal junction level. Superiorly, it can be followed to the origin of the superior hypogastric plexus.

Visceral pelvic fascia is formed from thickenings of connective tissue, which are closely associated with the pelvic viscera to which it relates and with the neurovascular structures related to those organs. In its most inferior and lateral extent, the visceral pelvic fascia is closely related to, and derives from, the superior fascia over the attachment of levator ani, whereas, more superiorly and posteriorly, it is derived from part of the piriformis fascia [1].

The visceral pelvic fascia covers the pelvic organs including prostate, bladder, and rectum. Therefore, visceral pelvic fascias composed of individual organ fasciae (e.g., rectal fascia, prostatic fascia) and connective sheets between pelvic organs (e.g., rectoprostatic or rectovaginal fasciae) or linking pelvic organs with pelvic walls (e.g., pubovesical ligaments). The pubovesical (or puboprostatic) ligaments are paired fibrous bands originating from visceral fascia, stretching from the posterior surface of the pubic bone adjacent, to the urethral sphincter, and to the ventral prostate. They stabilize the prostate, urethra, and urinary bladder representing a part of the "suspensory system" of the continence mechanisms.

On the lateral sidewalls of the pelvis, the parietal and the visceral pelvic fascia are fused at the level of the prostate and bladder; this fusion is named the fascial tendinous arch of the pelvis and extends from the pubovesical ligaments to the ischial spine. During surgery, access to the prostate may be gained by incision of the pelvic fascia either medial or lateral to this fusion. The incision of the pelvic fascia lateral to the tendinous arch of the pelvis leaves levator ani fascia adherent to the prostate and the levator ani muscle bare. Differently, when the pelvic fascia is incised medial to the tendinous arch, the levator ani fascia is not separated from the levator ani muscle fibers and the prostate remains covered only by its visceral (prostatic) fascia.

1.4   Perineum

The perineum is a diamond-shaped region located below the pelvic floor, between the inner aspects of the thighs and anterior to the sacrum and coccyx [1]. It is bounded anteriorly by the pubic symphysis and its arcuate ligament, posteriorly by the coccyx, anterolaterally by the ischiopubic rami and the ischial tuberosities, and posterolaterally by the sacrotuberous ligaments. The deep limit of the perineum is the inferior surface of the pelvic diaphragm and its superficial limit is the skin. A line drawn through the ischial tuberosities divides the perineum into an anal triangle, which faces downwards and backwards, and a urogenital triangle, that faces downwards and forwards.

Anal triangle is similar in males and females where the main difference is the wider transverse dimension of the triangle in females as a result of the larger size of the pelvic outlet. The anal triangle contains the anal canal with its sphincters and the ischioanal fossa with its contained nerves and vessels.

Urogenital triangle is posteriorly delimited by the interischial line which overlaps the posterior border of the transverse perineal muscles. Anteriorly and laterally, it is delimited by the symphysis pubis and ischiopubic rami. In males, the urogenital triangle expands superficially to the scrotum and to the root of the penis. In females, it extends to the lower limit of the labia and mons pubis. The urogenital triangle is divided into two parts by the perineal membrane, a triangular membrane attached laterally to the ischiopubic rami with its apex attached to the arcuate ligament of the pubis. *Deep perineal pouch* is bounded deeply by the inferior fascia of the pelvic floor and superficially by the perineal membrane. Between these two layers lie the deep transverse perinei, superficial to the urethral sphincter mechanism and pubourethralis, and in females superficial to the compressor urethrae and sphincter urethrovaginalis.

1.5   Pelvic Circulation (Arteries, Veins, Lymphatics)

1.5.1   Arteries

Common iliac arteries separate at the level of the sacroiliac joint into external and internal iliac arteries. *Internal iliac arteries* divide into an anterior trunk and a posterior trunk. Anterior to the artery is located the ureter and, in females, the ovary and fimbriated end of the uterine tube, while posterior to it are the internal iliac vein, the lumbosacral trunk, and the sacroiliac joint.

1.5.1.1 Posterior Trunk Branches

Iliolumbar artery ascends anterolaterally to the sacroiliac joint and lumbosacral nerve trunk. It lies posterior to the obturator nerve and external iliac vessels and reaches the medial border of psoas major [1] where it divides into the lumbar and iliac branches (Fig. 1.1). The former supplies psoas major and quadratus lumborum and then anastomoses with the fourth lumbar artery. The latter supplies iliacus and then anastomoses between with the iliac branches of the obturator artery. *Lateral sacral arteries* are usually double: the superior artery passes into the first/second anterior sacral foramen, supplies the sacral vertebrae, and then leaves to supply the skin and muscles dorsal to the sacrum. The *inferior sacral artery* crosses obliquely anterior to piriformis and the sacral anterior spinal rami and then descends lateral to the sympathetic trunk to anastomose with its fellow and the median sacral artery anterior to the coccyx. *Superior gluteal artery* is the largest branch of the internal

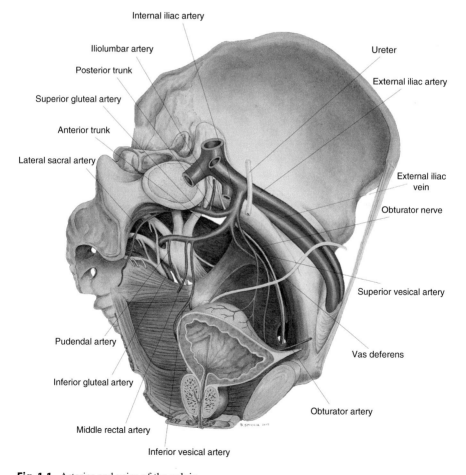

Internal iliac artery

Iliolumbar artery

Ureter

Posterior trunk

External iliac artery

Superior gluteal artery

Anterior trunk

Lateral sacral artery

External iliac vein

Obturator nerve

Superior vesical artery

Pudendal artery

Vas deferens

Inferior gluteal artery

Obturator artery

Middle rectal artery

Inferior vesical artery

Fig. 1.1 Arteries and veins of the pelvis

iliac artery and forms the main continuation of its posterior trunk. It runs posteriorly between the lumbosacral trunk and the first sacral ramus or between the first and second rami and then turns inferiorly, leaving the pelvis by the greater sciatic foramen above piriformis and dividing into superficial and deep branches where it supplies, in the pelvis, piriformis, and obturator internus (Fig. 1.1).

1.5.1.2 Anterior Trunk Branches

Superior vesical artery lies on the lateral wall of the pelvis just below the brim and runs anteroinferiorly medial to the periosteum of the posterior surface of the pubis (Fig. 1.1). It supplies the distal end of the ureter, the bladder, the proximal end of the vas deferens, and the seminal vesicles. *Inferior vesical artery* may arise as a common branch with the middle rectal artery. In the female, it is often replaced by the vaginal artery. It supplies the bladder, the prostate, the seminal vesicles, and the vas deferens. *Middle rectal artery* is often multiple and may be small. It runs into the lateral ligaments of the rectum. *Obturator artery* runs anteroinferiorly from the anterior trunk on the lateral pelvic wall to the upper part of the obturator foramen (Fig. 1.1). It leaves the pelvis via the obturator canal and divides into anterior and posterior branches. In the pelvis, it is related laterally to the fascia over obturator internus and is crossed on its medial aspect by the ureter and, in the male, by the vas deferens. The obturator nerve is above the artery, the obturator vein below it. *Uterine artery* is an additional branch in females and arises below the obturator artery on the lateral wall of the pelvis and runs inferomedially into the broad ligament of the uterus. *Internal pudendal artery* arises just below the origin of the obturator artery and it descends laterally to the inferior rim of the greater sciatic foramen, where it leaves the pelvis between piriformis and ischiococcygeus to enter the gluteal region (Fig. 1.1). *Inferior gluteal artery* descends posteriorly, anterior to the sacral plexus and piriformis but posterior to the internal pudendal artery (Fig. 1.1). Inside the pelvis, the inferior gluteal artery gives branches to piriformis, ischiococcygeus, and iliococcygeus and occasionally contributes to the middle rectal arterial supply.

External iliac arteries descend laterally along the medial border of psoas major, from the common iliac bifurcation to a point midway between the anterior superior iliac spine and the symphysis pubis, and enter the thigh posterior to the inguinal ligament to become the femoral artery.

1.5.2   Veins

Common iliac vein is formed by the union of the external and internal iliac veins, anterior to the sacroiliac joints.

Internal iliac vein is formed by the convergence of several veins above the greater sciatic foramen [1]. It ascends posteromedial to the internal iliac artery to join the external iliac vein, forming the common iliac vein at the pelvic brim, anterior to the lower part of the sacroiliac joint. It is covered anteromedially by parietal peritoneum. Its tributaries are: *Superior gluteal veins* are the venae comitantes of the superior gluteal artery and enter the pelvis via the greater sciatic foramen. *Inferior gluteal veins* are venae comitantes of the inferior gluteal artery. They begin proximally and posterior in the thigh, where they anastomose with the medial circumflex femoral and first perforating veins and enter the pelvis low in the greater sciatic foramen, joining to form a vessel opening into the distal part of the internal iliac vein. *Obturator vein* begins in the proximal adductor region and enters the pelvis via the obturator foramen. It runs posteriorly and superiorly on the lateral pelvic wall below the obturator artery and between the ureter and internal iliac artery and ends in the internal iliac vein. *Lateral sacral veins* run with the lateral sacral artery and are interconnected by a sacral venous plexus. *Middle rectal vein* begins in the rectal venous plexus, draining the rectum, and runs on the lateral pelvic surface of levator ani to end in the internal iliac vein.

External iliac vein is the proximal continuation of the femoral vein, posterior to the inguinal ligament, ending anterior to the sacroiliac joint where it joins the internal iliac vein to form the common iliac vein. On its left, it is medial to the external iliac artery as on the right side where it tends to lean behind it as the artery ascends. The external iliac vein is crossed medially by the ureter and internal iliac artery (Fig. 1.1). In males, it is crossed by the vas deferens and in females by the round ligament and ovarian vessels. It tributaries are *inferior epigastric vein*, *deep circumflex iliac vein*, and *pubic vein*.

1.5.3 Lymphatic Drainage

The pelvic lymph nodes are associated and accordingly named with the pelvic vessels around the common, external, and internal iliac arteries and veins. *Common iliac nodes* receive the entire lymphatic drainage of the lower limb draining both internal and external iliac nodes and lying in medial, lateral, and anterior chains around the common iliac artery. *External iliac nodes* are lateral, medial, and anterior to the external iliac vessels and receive the lymph from the lower limb, the glans penis or clitoris, the membranous urethra, prostate, fundus of the bladder, uterine cervix, and upper vagina. *Internal iliac nodes* surround the internal iliac vessels and receive the lymph from the pelvic viscera, the deeper parts of the perineum, and the gluteal and posterior femoral muscles.

1.6 Pelvic Innervation

The posterior abdominal wall contains the origin of the lumbar plexus and numerous autonomic plexuses and ganglia, which lie close to the abdominal aorta and its branches. The lumbar ventral rami descend laterally into psoas major and increase in size from first to last. The first three and most of the fourth form the lumbar plexus; the smaller moiety of the fourth joins the fifth as a lumbosacral trunk, which joins the sacral plexus.

The pelvis contains the lumbosacral nerve trunk, the sacral and coccygeal plexuses, and the pelvic parts of the sympathetic and parasympathetic systems

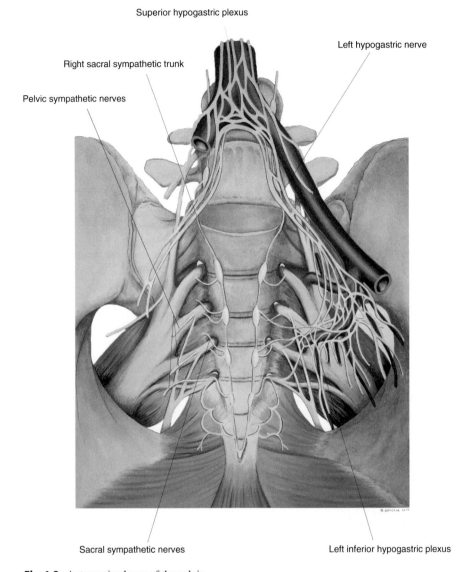

Superior hypogastric plexus

Left hypogastric nerve

Right sacral sympathetic trunk

Pelvic sympathetic nerves

Sacral sympathetic nerves

Left inferior hypogastric plexus

Fig. 1.2 Autonomic plexus of the pelvis

(Fig. 1.2). Collectively, these nerves carry the somatic and autonomic innervation to the majority of the pelvic visceral organs, the pelvic floor and perineum, the gluteal region, and the lower limb. The ventral rami of the sacral and coccygeal spinal nerves form the sacral and coccygeal plexuses. The first and second sacral ventral rami are large, the third to fifth diminish progressively, and the coccygeal is the smallest. Each receives a gray ramus communicans from a corresponding sympathetic ganglion. Visceral efferent rami leave the second to fourth sacral rami as the pelvic splanchnic nerves, containing parasympathetic fibers to minute ganglia in the walls of the pelvic viscera.

1.6.1   Lumbar Plexus

The lumbar plexus lies within the substance of the posterior part of psoas major, anterior to the transverse processes of the lumbar vertebrae and in "line" with the intervertebral foramina. It is formed by the first three, and most of the fourth, lumbar ventral rami, with a contribution from the 12th thoracic ventral ramus. The first lumbar ventral ramus, joined by a branch from the 12th thoracic ventral ramus, bifurcates, and the upper and larger part divides again into the iliohypogastric and ilioinguinal nerves. The smaller lower part unites with a branch from the second lumbar ventral ramus to form the genitofemoral nerve. The remainder of the second, third, and part of the fourth lumbar ventral rami join the plexus and divide into ventral and dorsal branches. Ventral branches of the second to fourth rami join to form the obturator nerve. The main dorsal branches of the second to fourth rami join to form the femoral nerve. Small branches from the dorsal branches of the second and third rami join to form the lateral femoral cutaneous nerve. The accessory obturator nerve, when it exists, arises from the third and fourth ventral branches. The lumbar plexus is supplied by branches from the lumbar vessels which supply psoas major. *Iliohypogastric nerve* travels and divides between internal oblique and transversus muscles into lateral and anterior cutaneous branches, supplying both muscles. The first branch runs through internal and external oblique above the iliac crest and supplies the posterolateral gluteal skin. The second cutaneous branch runs through internal oblique approximately 2 cm medial to the anterior superior iliac spine and through the external oblique aponeurosis 3 cm above the superficial inguinal ring, distributing to the internal oblique and transversus abdominis and supplying sensation over the lower anterior abdomen and pubis. *Ilioinguinal nerve* passes across quadratus lumborum and the upper part of iliacus obliquely and, close to the anterior end of the iliac crest, enters transversus abdominis. It pierces and supplies the internal oblique muscle and then passes the inguinal canal below the spermatic cord emerging from the external inguinal ring to provide sensation to the mons pubis and anterior scrotum or labia majora. *Genitofemoral nerve* pierces the psoas muscle to reach its anterior surface in the retroperitoneum and then travels to the pelvis and splits into genital and femoral branches. The genital branch crosses the lower part of the external iliac artery, enters the inguinal canal by the internal ring, and supplies cremaster and the skin of the scrotum in males. In females, it accompanies the round ligament and ends in the skin of the mons pubis and labium majus. The femoral branch descends lateral to the external iliac artery and crosses the deep circumflex iliac artery, passing behind the inguinal ligament and entering the femoral sheath lateral to the femoral artery. It pierces the anterior layer of the femoral sheath and fascia lata and supplies the skin anterior to the upper part of the femoral triangle.

Femoral nerve descends through psoas major and then exits its lateral side to pass under the inguinal ligament. *Lateral femoral cutaneous nerve* of the thigh emerges from the lateral border of psoas major and crosses iliacus obliquely towards the anterior superior iliac spine. The right nerve passes posterolateral to the caecum, while the left nerve passes behind the lower part of the descending colon. Both nerves pass behind or through the inguinal ligament into the thigh. *Obturator nerve* emerges in the true pelvis from beneath the psoas muscle, lateral to the internal iliac vessels, and passes through the obturator fossa to the obturator canal (Fig. 1.2). It descends on the lateral wall of the pelvis attached to the fascia over obturator internus and lies anterosuperior to the obturator vessels before running into the obturator foramen to enter the thigh. *Accessory obturator nerve*, when present, emerges from the medial border of psoas major and runs along this border over the posterior surface of the superior pubic ramus posterior to pectineus. It gives off branches here to supply pectineus and the hip joint.

1.6.1.1 Lumbosacral Trunk and Sacral Plexus

The sacral plexus is composed by the lumbosacral trunk, the first to third sacral ventral rami and part of the fourth sacral ventral ramus. The lumbar part of the lumbosacral trunk includes part of the fourth and all the fifth lumbar ventral rami and starts at the medial margin of psoas muscle and descends over the pelvic brim joining the first sacral ramus. The second and third sacral rami converge on the inferomedial aspect of the lumbosacral trunk in the greater sciatic foramen to create the sciatic nerve. The sacral plexus lies on the pelvic surface of the piriformis deep to the endopelvic fascia and posterior to the internal iliac vessels. It leaves the pelvis through the greater sciatic foramen immediately posterior to the sacrospinous ligament and supplies motor and sensory innervation to the posterior thigh and lower leg.

1.6.1.2 Pelvic Autonomic Plexus and Neurovascular Bundle (NVB)

The presynaptic sympathetic cell bodies reside in the lateral column of gray matter, in the last three thoracic and first two lumbar segments of the spinal cord, reaching the pelvic plexus by two pathways: (1) the superior hypogastric plexus is formed by sympathetic fibers from the celiac plexus and the first four lumbar splanchnic nerves, and it divides, anterior to the bifurcation of the aorta, into two hypogastric nerves that enter the pelvis medial to the internal iliac vessels, anteriorly to the sacrum, and deep to the endopelvic fascia and (2) the pelvic continuations of the sympathetic trunks pass deep to the common iliac vessels and medial to the sacral foramina and fuse in front of the coccyx at the ganglion impar. Each chain comprises four to five ganglia that send branches anterolaterally in order to create the pelvic plexus. Presynaptic parasympathetic innervation arises from the intermediolateral cell column of the sacral cord. Fibers emerge from the second, third, and fourth sacral spinal nerves as the nervi erigentes to join the hypogastric nerves.

Sympathetic and parasympathetic components merge to form the pelvic plexus (or inferior hypogastric plexus) (Fig. 1.2), which is oriented in the sagittal plane on either side between the rectum and the urinary bladder. In the male, the pelvic plexus is responsible for the mechanisms of erection, ejaculation, and urinary continence. Sympathetic fibers derive from the hypogastric nerve and are responsible for ejaculation; parasympathetic fibers, including nervi erigentes, derive from the pelvic and sacral splanchnic nerves.

Branches of the pelvic plexus follow pelvic blood vessels to reach the pelvic viscera. The distal portion of the pelvic plexus innervates the prostate and the cavernosal nerves [3].

Fibers of the pelvic plexus are mostly located at the lateral side of pelvic organs (bladder neck, prostate, and the seminal vesicles) arranged in a cage-like fashion, whereas few fibers are found on the anterior surfaces of these organs. These nerves are hardly identifiable during surgical procedures. Interestingly, cavernous nerves, branches of the pelvic plexus, run close to the posterolateral surface and tips of the seminal vesicles and could be preserved by the accurate dissection of seminal vesicles during radical prostatectomy, thus reducing the degree and risk of postoperative complications [4]. From here, the pelvic plexus and cavernous nerves continue inferiorly and reach the lateral surface of the prostate. Here, the nervous fibers remain microscopic and are accompanied by vascular vessels; this complex of microscopic nerves and vessels is named neurovascular bundle (NVB). NVB provide innervation and blood supply to prostate; thus, its branches penetrate into the prostate capsule and tether the NVB to prostate. The organization of NVB is complex and disordered and its preservation (nerve-sparing procedure) represents a surgical challenge [5].

1.7 Pelvic Organs

1.7.1 Pelvic Ureter

The ureter is divided into abdominal and pelvic parts by the common iliac artery. The ureter is identified intraoperatively by its peristaltic waves and is found anterior to the bifurcation of the common iliac artery (Fig. 1.3). Once the ureters enter the pelvis, they spread along the pelvic sidewalls towards the ischial spines, then turning anteriorly and medially to reach the bladder. In males, the ureter is crossed anteriorly by the vas deferens and runs with the inferior vesical arteries, veins, and nerves in the lateral vesical ligaments. In females, the ureter passes medial to the ovarian vessels and then posterior to the uterine artery within the cardinal ligament. The ureter courses 1–4 cm on the anterior vaginal wall to reach the bladder [2]. Occasionally, a stone lodged in the distal ureter can be palpated through the anterior vaginal wall [2].

The ureter receives its blood supply from the common iliac artery and internal iliac artery through the inferior vesical and uterine arteries, and they all enter laterally to the pelvic ureter; thus the peritoneum should be incised medially to avoid injury to its blood supply. Lymphatic Drainage is through external, internal, and common iliac lymph nodes; thus pathologic enlargement of these lymph nodes can obstruct the ureter. Innervation is from the hypogastric nerve and inferior hypogastric plexus.

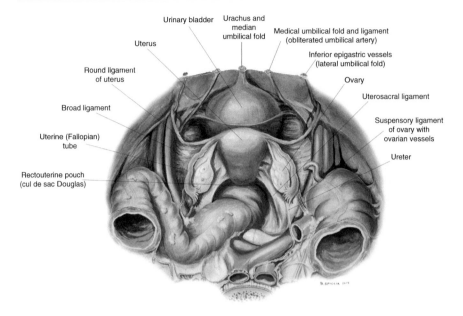

Fig. 1.3 Female pelvic cavity and contents

1.7.2   Urinary Bladder

The bladder acts as a reservoir; it is a pelvic organ when empty and an abdominal organ when full, displacing the parietal peritoneum from the suprapubic region to make it possible to perform a suprapubic cystostomy without risking the entrance into the peritoneal cavity. Superiorly it is covered by peritoneum and has the median umbilical ligament (urachus) (Fig. 1.4) that extends from the apex to the umbilicus covered by the peritoneum to form the median umbilical fold. In males, posteriorly, the peritoneum separates it from the rectum forming the rectovesical pouch of Douglas (Fig. 1.4). Anteriorly it is separated from the transversalis fascia by fat in the space of Retzius that is an extraperitoneal space separating it from the pubic symphysis; this space provides access to the prostate during laparoscopic radical prostatectomy. In females, the peritoneum separates the uterus from the bladder through vesicouterine pouch superiorly and the uterus from the rectum through rectouterine pouch (of Douglas) (Fig. 1.3), posteriorly. At the bladder neck, the detrusor muscle forms the internal sphincter which is responsible of continence and, in cases of destroyed striated sphincter, it can maintain continence. This sphincter has abundant adrenergic receptors that close the bladder neck during ejaculation, and damage to the sympathetic nerves to the bladder, as a result of diabetes mellitus or retroperitoneal lymph node dissection, can cause retrograde ejaculation. In females, the bladder neck has limited sphincter function and little adrenergic receptors. The bladder is fixed inferiorly by thickenings of pelvic fascia attaching it to rectum, pelvic sidewalls, and pubic bone. The pubovesical ligaments extend from the bladder neck to the pubic bones; in females they constitute the pubourethral ligaments,

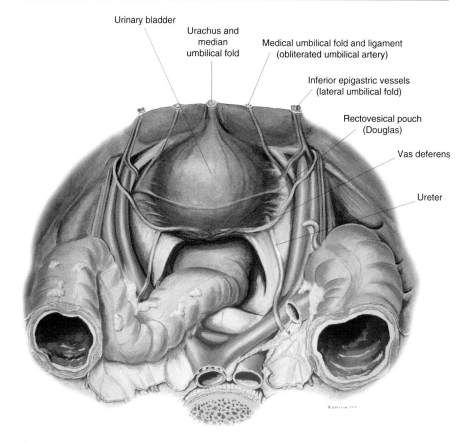

Fig. 1.4 Male pelvic cavity and contents

while in males they constitute the puboprostatic ligaments. The bladder base has lateral and posterior ligaments in males; the lateral ligaments are the peritoneal reflections from the bladder to the pelvic sidewalls, while the posterior ligaments are the sacrogenital folds. In females, these ligaments are equivalent to cardinal and uterosacral ligaments (Fig. 1.3). Anterior to the bladder, there are three peritoneal folds on the abdominal wall: (1) median umbilical fold covering the median umbilical ligament (urachus), (2) two medial umbilical folds covering the medial umbilical ligaments (obliterated umbilical arteries) (Fig. 1.4), and (3) two lateral umbilical folds covering the inferior epigastric vessels (Fig. 1.3).

The bladder is supplied by the superior and inferior vesical arteries from the internal iliac artery; it is also supplied by obturator, inferior gluteal, uterine, and vaginal arteries. Vesical veins join to form vesical plexus that drains into the internal iliac vein. Lymphatic drainage is mainly to external iliac lymph nodes and the remaining into obturator, internal iliac, and common iliac lymph nodes. Autonomic efferent fibers from the anterior portion of the pelvic plexus (the vesical plexus) pass up the lateral and posterior ligaments to innervate the bladder.

1.7.3   Prostate

The prostate has an anterior, posterior, and lateral surfaces with an apex inferiorly and a base superiorly contagious with the bladder base. On the apex, the puboprostatic ligaments fix it to the pubic bones anteriorly. Anterolaterally, the prostatic capsule intermingles with the endopelvic fascia. The superficial branch of the dorsal vein lies outside this fascia in the retropubic fat and pierces it to drain into the dorsal vein complex. Laterally the prostate is related to the levator ani muscle and fascia (Fig. 1.5). The prostate is covered by a fibrous capsule; external to prostate capsule, a series of fascias are present and collectively called periprostatic fascias.

In accordance with their location, the periprostatic fascias can be divided into three elements: the anterior, the lateral, and the posterior fascias. The anterior periprostatic fascia is associated with the anterior surface of the prostate and covers the so-called dorsal vascular complex, a venous plexus which drains blood from penile and urethral veins and contains small arteries from the inferior vesical artery. The lateral periprostatic fascia is disposed on the lateral surfaces of the prostate; it is composed of an external layer which corresponds to the levator ani fascia and an inner layer which is called the prostatic fascia. The prostatic fascia is a sheet of connective tissue covering

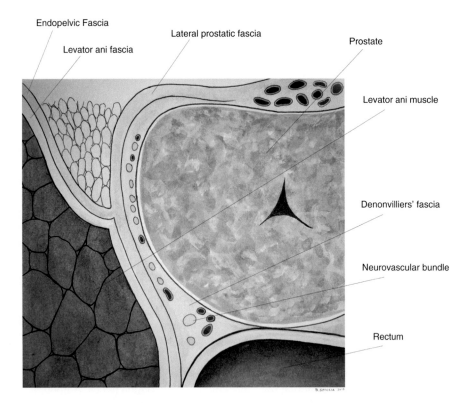

Fig. 1.5 Prostatic fascial layers

the prostate capsule and extending from the anterior to the posterior surfaces of the prostate. Interestingly, prostatic fascia passes medial to the NVB, while the levator ani fascia remains lateral. From a surgical point of view, the prostatic fascia forms an intrafascial plane between the fascia and the prostate capsule, while the levator ani fascia serves as the boundary for the interfascial plane. The prostatic fascia continues on the posterior surface of the prostate as posterior-prostatic fascia and is in continuity with the seminal vesicle fascia forming the so-called Denonvilliers' fascia (or recto-prostatic fascia). Superiorly, the Denonvilliers' fascia corresponds to the caudal end of the rectovesical pouch; inferiorly, it ends at the level of prostate-urethral junction in continuity with the central perineal tendon. Posteriorly, the Denonvilliers' fascia is covered by the thin rectal fascia. Anteriorly, the Denonvilliers' fascia is often fused with prostate capsule at the center of the posterior-prostatic surface; proceeding laterally, the Denonvilliers' fascia does not adhere to the prostatic capsule and the space between the fascia and the prostatic capsule is occupied by areolar tissue and NVB elements. Interestingly, no NVB elements are found lateral to levator ani fascia and posterior to the Denonvilliers' fascia [6].

The prostate is made of 70 % glands and 30 % fibromuscular stroma and has five lobes: anterior, posterior, median, and two lateral lobes. The glandular part has three zones: peripheral (70 %), central (25 %), and transitional (5 %) zones. The transitional zone is separated from the other zones by a thin fibromuscular band that gets compressed by benign prostatic hyperplasia arising from this zone to form the surgical capsule that is seen during prostate enucleation, and it accounts for 20 % of prostatic adenocarcinomas. 1–5 % of prostatic adenocarcinomas arise from the central zone, while the majority (70 %) of them arise from the peripheral zone that is also the most common site of chronic prostatitis. The urethra traverses the prostate becoming the prostatic urethra that is divided into proximal and distal parts; it is lined by transitional epithelium.

The prostate is supplied by the inferior vesical artery that gives two branches: urethral and capsular branches; the venous drainage is to the periprostatic plexus that receives tributaries from the deep dorsal vein of the penis (mainly) and vesical veins to drain into the internal iliac vein. The lymphatic drainage is mainly to the obturator and internal iliac lymph nodes with little drainage to the external iliac lymph nodes. Sympathetic and parasympathetic innervation from the pelvic (inferior hypogastric) plexus travels to the prostate through the cavernous nerves, sympathetic causes smooth muscle contraction and parasympathetic causes secretion.

1.7.4 Membranous Urethra

It is the least dilatable, narrowest, and the shortest (2–2.5 cm) part of the urethra. It extends from the apex of prostate to the perineal membrane. The wall of the membranous urethra consists of intrinsic smooth muscle part which is involuntary under autonomic control and extrinsic striated muscle part which is under voluntary control, and both parts form the external urethral sphincter. Urine continence at this level is mediated by (1) radial folds of the pseudostratified columnar epithelium of urethral mucosa, (2) submucosal connective tissue, (3) intrinsic smooth muscle, (4) extrinsic striated muscle, and (5) puborectalis component of levator ani. The striated external urethral sphincter has a posterior fibrous defect and is inserted throughout its length into the perineal body; thus when the sphincter contracts, the urethral walls are pulled towards the perineal body to seal the urethra. The striated sphincter is surrounded by the dorsal vein complex anteriorly, levator ani laterally, and recto-urethralis and the perineal body posteriorly and is suspended anteriorly to the suspensory ligament of penis and posteriorly to the puboprostatic ligament from its anterior and lateral parts. Two bulbourethral glands are invested in sphincteric muscle and drain into the membranous urethra during sexual excitement.

The striated sphincter has two sources of nerve supply: (1) pudendal nerve and (2) pelvic floor somatic efferent nerves from sacral plexus. Injury to this nerve at radical prostatectomy may contribute to postoperative urinary incontinence [7]. The intrinsic smooth muscle is autonomically innervated by cavernous nerve.

1.7.5   Vas Deferens and Seminal Vesicles

The vas begins from the tail of epididymis (scrotal or testicular part) and is 45 cm long; initially it is very tortuous for 2–3 cm then straights up as it ascends in the posterior part of the spermatic cord (funicular or spermatic part) and through the inguinal canal (inguinal part). At the internal inguinal ring, it leaves the cord to enter the pelvis (pelvic part, longest) lateral to the inferior epigastric vessels (Fig. 1.4) and passes medial to all the pelvic sidewall structures reaching base of the prostate posteriorly where it joins the seminal vesicle duct forming the ejaculatory duct. The ampulla of the vas is seen posterior to the bladder where its lumen becomes dilated and tortuous and it is capable of storing spermatozoa.

The seminal vesicle is a single coiled tube that contributes to 85 % of seminal fluid volume and is found lateral to the vas and posterior to the bladder; both the vas and seminal vesicles are separated from the rectum by Denonvilliers' fascia, posteriorly.

The vas and seminal vesicles are supplied by vesiculo-deferential artery, a branch of superior vesical artery. During radical prostatectomy, this artery is encountered between the vas and seminal vesicle which should be ligated to avoid bleeding. Venous drainage is to the pelvic venous plexus and lymphatic drainage is to the external and internal iliac lymph nodes; they are innervated by sympathetic fibers from the pelvic plexus.

1.7.6   Uterus, Cervix, and Ovary

The uterus is found in the pelvis posterior to the bladder and uterovesical space and anterior to the rectum and rectouterine space. It is divided into (1) cervix, (2) body (corpus), and (3) fundus. The fallopian tubes extend laterally from the junction of the body and fundus and are divided into (1) uterine, (2) isthmus, (3) ampulla, and (4) infundibulum. The broad ligament is a two-layered folds of peritoneum that connects the sides of the uterus to the pelvic sidewalls and floor and is divided into (1) mesometrium, (2) mesosalpinx, and (3) mesovarium.

The ovary is found posterior to the tube and has two ligaments; the ligament of ovary fixes it to the lateral wall of the uterus, while the suspensory ligament of ovary (infundibulopelvic ligament) fixes it to the pelvic sidewalls carrying the ovarian vessels with it (Fig. 1.3). The round ligament originates at the uterine horns, leaves the pelvis through the internal inguinal ring passing through the inguinal canal, and attaches to labial fat pad (Fig. 1.3). The cardinal ligament attaches the cervix to the pelvic sidewalls by attaching to the obturator fascia; on the other hand, the uterosacral ligament attaches the uterus to the sacrum (Fig. 1.3).

The uterine artery passes in front of the ureter running in the cardinal and broad ligaments and gives branches to supply the vagina, uterus, and fallopian tubes. During hysterectomy, great care must be taken during isolation and ligation of uterine artery to avoid injuring the ureter. The uterine veins run adjacent to the arteries and drain to the internal iliac vein, the uterine venous plexus anastomoses with the vaginal and ovarian venous plexuses. Lymphatic drainage is to external iliac, internal iliac and obturator lymph nodes, innervation is mainly by pelvic plexus. The nerves and vessels travel through the cardinal and uterosacral ligaments to supply the female pelvic organs, and during hysterectomy, it can lead to atonic neurogenic bladder.

References

1. Susan Standring and Editorial Board. Gray's anatomy. The anatomical basis of clinical practice, Chruchill Livingstone Elsevier, Fortieth edition, UK 2008.
2. Alan JW, Louis RK, Alan WP, Craig AP. Campbell-Walsh Urology, 11th ed. 2016.
3. Park YH, Jeong CW, Lee SE. A comprehensive review of neuroanatomy of the prostate. Prostate Int. 2013;1:139–45.
4. Walz J, Burnett AL, Costello AJ, Eastham JA, Graefen M, Guillonneau B, et al. A critical analysis of the current knowledge of surgical anatomy related to optimization of cancer control and preservation of continence and erection in candidates for radical prostatectomy. Eur Urol. 2010;57:179–92.
5. Costello AJ, Brooks M, Cole OJ. Anatomical studies of the neurovascular bundle and cavernosal nerves. BJU Int. 2004;94:1071–6.
6. Lindsey I, Guy RJ, Warren BF, et al. Anatomy of Denonvilliers' fascia and pelvic nerves, impotence, and implications for the colorectal surgeon. Br J Surg. 2000;87:1288–99.
7. Hollabaugh RS, Dmochowski RR, Steiner MS. Neuroanatomy of the male rhabdosphincter. Urology. 1997;49:426–34.

Preoperative Assessment and Intraoperative Anesthesiologic Care in Mini-Invasive Laparoscopic Surgery

2

Flaminia Coluzzi, Thomas J. Pallaria, Anand Thakur, and Joseph Pergolizzi

2.1   General Anesthesia for Laparoscopic Procedures

Laparoscopic surgery is an established technique for minimally invasive surgery of the chest, abdomen, and pelvis, and it has been used in several surgical disciplines. Its early application was in gynecological surgery in the 1960s and 1970s. Laparoscopic surgery appeared to be advantageous compared to open, chest, abdominal, and pelvic surgery in reducing surgical trauma, lessening postoperative pulmonary complications, decreasing both postoperative pain, and ileus, allowing earlier ambulation and improving recovery times. From an economic standpoint these minimally invasive procedures decrease hospital stay and provide an earlier return to everyday activities. The disadvantages include longer anesthesia and surgical times, a steeper learning curve, and higher equipment costs.

Laparoscopic surgery is most commonly performed under general anesthesia with an endotracheal tube and controlled mechanical ventilation with American Society of Anaesthesiology (ASA) standard monitoring. Anesthetic goals during laparoscopic surgery are as follows: decompression of the gastrointestinal tract with either

F. Coluzzi (✉)
Department of Medico-Surgical Sciences and Biotechnologies, Unit of Anaesthesia, Intensive Care and Pain Medicine, Sapienza University of Rome, Rome, Italy
e-mail: flaminia.coluzzi@uniroma1.it

T.J. Pallaria
Department of Anesthesiology, Newark Beth Israel Medical Center – Rutgers University School of Medline, New Brunswick, NJ, USA

A. Thakur
Department of Anesthesiology, Wayne State University, Detroit, MI, USA

J. Pergolizzi, MD
Temple University School of Medicine, Philadelphia, PA, USA

Johns Hopkins University School of Medicine, Baltimore, MD, USA

© Springer International Publishing Switzerland 2016   21
A. Carbone et al. (eds.), *Functional Urologic Surgery in Neurogenic and Oncologic Diseases*, Urodynamics, Neurourology and Pelvic Floor Dysfunctions, DOI 10.1007/978-3-319-29191-8_2

an orogastric tube or nasogastric tube, adequate skeletal muscle relaxation, management of the effects of pneumoperitoneum (resulting from the insufflation of carbon dioxide (CO_2)), and Trendelenburg positioning with appropriate patient padding and positioning. These measures are designed to obtain an adequate exposure of the surgical field decreasing potential surgical trauma and intraoperative injury to the patient. The anesthetic goals are to improve surgical conditions optimizing the physiological response to cardiovascular, pulmonary, and CNS functioning; these conditions facilitate the surgeon to potentially decrease operative time and trauma [1].

2.1.1   Preoperative Evaluation for General Anesthesia

The preoperative anesthetic evaluation of patients undergoing laparoscopic surgery involves a careful history and physical examination, focusing particularly on the airway as to predict difficult tracheal intubation (Mallampati classification). In addition body mass index (BMI), medications, allergies, and patient position for the specific laparoscopic surgical procedure have to be considered.

2.1.1.1 Is the Patient Eligible to Undergo Laparoscopic Surgery?

A complete history and physical evaluation with careful examination of the airway, ASA status, paying particular attention to the optimization of cardiovascular and respiratory functioning, are necessary to determine whether the patient is eligible for laparoscopic surgery. The ASA physical status looks at the health condition of the patient classifying him/her from class I to class V, class I being the most healthy and medically optimized and class V being the higher surgical medical risk with highest chance of poor potential outcome or demise [2].

Cardiovascular and Respiratory Assessment

Cardiovascular assessment of the patient for laparoscopic surgery involves a detailed history and physical outlining, hypertension, arrhythmia, heart disease and failure, previous heart attack, recent chest pain, and/or stroke-like symptoms, high cholesterol. It also involves observing the patient's cardiovascular tolerance to activity, from regular to strenuous exercise. While the electrocardiogram (EKG) is mandatory in every patients, echo or stress test, Holter, arrhythmia monitoring, cardiac magnetic resonance imaging (MRI), or cardiac catheterization with emphasis on cardiac perfusion status and ejection fraction should be performed only if indicated. These results help in quantifying evidence of heart disease and functional ability of the heart.

Pulmonary assessment of the patient for laparoscopic surgery involves a detailed history and physical outlining, smoking and tobacco use habit, shortness of breath, orthopnea, dyspnea, chest pain, asthma, bronchitis, chronic obstructive pulmonary disease (COPD), and emphysema. Testing for pulmonary status can involve chest x-ray and pulmonary function tests including the evaluation of patient's respiratory functional status with the use of inhalers or supplemental oxygen, exercise tolerance, and carbon monoxide diffusion testing.

These tests can help quantify evidence of pulmonary disease and functional ability of the lungs.

Usually a careful history and physical examination with emphasis on exercise tolerance evaluation of metabolic equivalents (METs) and the use of medications will give us enough information without further extensive testing.

2.1.2 Intraoperative Management for General Anesthesia

2.1.2.1 Effects of Positioning (Cardiovascular and Respiratory)

In the anatomical supine position, cardiac output (CO) and venous return are generally maintained. In the Trendelenburg position (head down), generally venous return and CO increase. During urological laparoscopy, despite the Trendelenburg position, venous return and CO are generally decreased, due to the addition of carbon dioxide in a pneumoperitoneum [3].

When the patient is placed in prolonged extreme Trendelenburg position with a pneumoperitoneum, a precipitous decrease in venous return from the head may result. This can lead to increased intracranial and intraocular pressures, thus causing cerebral edema and retinal detachment. Decreased venous return and venous stasis can also lead to cyanosis and edema in the face and neck.

Respiratory effects of the Trendelenburg position (a tilt of 20–30°) include decreased functional residual capacity (FRC), atelectasis, ventilation perfusion (V/Q) mismatch, and potential hypoxemia and hypercarbia. Positive end-expiratory pressure (PEEP) may be used to increase intraoperative FRC and reduce intraoperative hypoxemia and postoperative atelectasis.

Two other positions with physiologic impact are the reverse Trendelenburg (head up) and the lithotomy position. The reverse Trendelenburg position reduces venous return, which may lead to decrease in cardiac output and mean arterial pressure. The lithotomy position will induce autotransfusion by augmenting blood from vessels of the lower extremities into the central body compartment, which will consequently increase the venous return and preload to the heart.

2.1.2.2 Effects of Pneumoperitoneum (Cardiovascular and Respiratory)

Hemodynamic disturbances during laparoscopy are commonly the result of insufflation of the abdomen with carbon dioxide and pneumoperitoneum. Normal intra-abdominal pressure (IAP) is 0–5 mmHg. The pneumoperitoneum is created by insufflating the abdomen with pressures of 15–20 mmHg. Increases in IAP greater than 10 mmHg manifest themselves clinically, and IAP greater than 15 mmHg can potentially result in an abdominal compartment syndrome, which affects multiple organ systems [4].

The cardiovascular effects of pneumoperitoneum can be understood via the following simple mathematical relationship, which expresses determinants of mean arterial pressure:

$$\text{Mean Arterial Pressure (MAP)} = \text{Cardiac Output (CO)} \times \text{Systemic Vascular Resistance (SVR)}$$

Even though pneumoperitoneum causes an increase in SVR while causing a decrease in CO, an overall MAP increase is witnessed because raising values of SVR exceed CO reduction.

These effects are proportional to the increase in IAP. The cause for increased SVR is the distention of the peritoneum and compression of the abdominal organs and blood vessels. Resistance to flow through arterial beds is increased due to both mechanical (distention and compression as mentioned above) and concomitant neurohumoral factors (e.g., release of catecholamines and vasopressin and activation of the renin-angiotensin system as a function of decreased venous return and decreased preload).

The pneumoperitoneum causes a decrease in CO for a number of reasons: (1) the decreased venous return (i.e., decreased cardiac preload) from compression of the inferior vena cava; (2) the increased resistance in venous circulation; and (3) hypovolemia due to possible preoperative bowel preparation and perioperative n.p.o. (*nihil* per os) status. CO typically reduces from 10 % to 30 %. However, despite a decrease in intracardiac blood volume, intracardiac filling pressures may be elevated due to the pressure transmitted across the diaphragm to the heart. Analogous effects in the pulmonary circulation manifest themselves as an increase in pulmonary vascular resistance (PVR) and decrease in CO to the lungs.

Healthy patients appear to tolerate these hemodynamic effects well. Several studies show that end-organ perfusion is maintained in these patients despite a decrease in CO. However, patients with cardiac disease may be exposed to an increased risk for further cardiac impairment. Patients with intravascular volume depletion appear worse to tolerate these effects. To minimize these effects, the lowest insufflation pressure required to achieve adequate surgical exposure should be used. Deep neuromuscular block during laparoscopy may be useful to reduce the pressure of pneumoperitoneum and to optimize abdominal space. Ideally, insufflation pressure should be less than 15 mmHg. Increases in SVR may be treated with vasodilating agents, centrally acting alpha-2 agonists or opioids. Decreases in venous return and CO may be attenuated by appropriate intravenous fluid loading prior to the induction of pneumoperitoneum.

Pneumoperitoneum may alter renal function (reduced renal cortex and medullary blood flow, decreased glomerular filtration and creatinine clearance), thus reducing urine output. Mannitol and furosemide may be used to force urine flow.

During radical prostatectomy, extraperitoneal insufflation may be intentional; however, carbon dioxide subcutaneous emphysema can develop as a complication. Carbon dioxide is readily absorbed, causing respiratory acidosis. Retroperitoneal insufflation may cause a major accumulation of CO_2.

Close monitoring of the end-tidal CO_2 is required during the whole procedure performed under general anesthesia. Laparoscopic surgery may require the routine use of blood gas analysis for monitoring respiratory function, particularly in frail patients or when procedures last more than 2 h.

2.2   Central Blocks for Urological Endoscopic Procedures

Spinal anesthesia involves the injection of local anesthetic (with or without opioids) into the subarachnoid space, resulting in an interruption of neural transmission impulses due to a conduction blockade of the spinal nerves, providing surgical anesthesia in the regions from the upper abdomen to the lowest peripheral anatomy. The susceptibility to local anesthetics is dependent upon the type of nerve fibers that are being targeted for blockade. These nerve fibers, which vary in diameter, thickness of the surrounding myelin sheath, and function, are more easily blocked according to how permeable they are to the local anesthetic. The smaller, preganglionic B fibers, for instance, are easier to be blocked than the larger sensory C fibers. The blockades achieved will be sensory, motor, and sympathetic-altering. Sympathetic blockade will occur one to two segments above the level of sensory blockade, and motor blockade will occur one to two segments below the level of sensory blockade. The subarachnoid injection of local anesthetic can be a single injection or through an indwelling catheter to allow repeated doses to be delivered during a surgical procedure [5].

2.2.1   Preoperative Evaluation for Spinal Anesthesia

The preoperative evaluation for a patient undergoing a surgical procedure receiving a central block is consistent with those who will be receiving a general anesthetic. The same vigilance in the history and physical assessment and airway classification must occur. The advantages of the subarachnoid blockade (SAB) over the use of a general anesthetic are to minimize the metabolic stress response to the procedure in patients with various comorbidities, to minimize intraoperative blood loss and/or the incidence of venous thromboembolic complications, and to allow an ongoing intraoperative neurologic assessment to identify developing symptoms of transurethral resection of the prostate (TURP) syndrome, a collection of symptoms caused by excessive intravascular absorption of the irrigating solution, such as restlessness, confusion, and nausea [6].

Although these advantages exist for the use of SAB, absolute and relative contraindications must be considered prior to deciding between general anesthesia and SAB.

Absolute contraindications are patient refusal, allergy to local anesthetics, increased intracranial pressure (ICP), unstable central nervous system disease, infection at needle insertion site, septicemia/bacteremia, severe hypovolemia, severe stenotic valvular heart disease, symmetrical septal hypertrophy, bleeding diathesis such as genetic (hemophilia) and acquired (disseminated intravascular coagulation – DIC), and patients receiving anticoagulation therapy.

The absolute contraindications related to blood clotting processes are due to the associated risks of spinal hematoma, which may lead to acute and or permanent neurologic dysfunction. Because of these risks, a coagulation assessment should be included in the preoperative evaluation and may include one or more of the following: platelet count, bleeding time, activated clotting time (ACT), platelet aggregation test, prothrombin time (PT), partial thromboplastin time (PTT), and international normalized ratio (INR) [7].

Relative contraindications are chronic headache/backache, severe deformities of the spinal column, untreated chronic hypertension, and minor abnormalities in blood clotting secondary to chronic aspirin therapy [6].

2.2.2   Intraoperative Management for Spinal Anesthesia

Once preoperative assessment and surgical considerations have determined that regional anesthesia is the optimal choice for the patient, technique and pharmacologic management of the SAB must be determined.

Placement of a SAB occurs in three principle positions: sitting, prone, and lateral decubitus. Maximal identification of midline and interspaces, baricity of the local anesthetic, the patient's comorbidities, and his/her body habitus will have a factor in determining the optimal position.

A typical SAB is performed in the lumbar region below the level of the spinal cord (L2-L3-L4) which should provide anesthesia to a dermatome level of the umbilicus (T10). Various types and sizes of needles are available for the lumbar puncture, with a standard length of 3.5″ (90 mm) and diameter ranges of 22–27 gauge (0.7–0.4 mm). The types of needle tips utilized are typically chosen based upon provider familiarity and preference. Types of tips available are cutting (Quincke) and pencil point (Sprotte and Whitacre), all beveled designed to puncture the dura with a minimal degree of post-puncture cerebral spinal fluid (CSF) leakage [8].

The level of spinal anaesthesia is dependent on the choice of local anesthetic, the dose administered, and its distribution within the subarachnoid space. Potency of local anesthetics is related to lipid solubility. The volume of the solution injected, the preexisting volume of the spinal subarachnoid space, the rate of the injection, and the effects of gravity determine the spread of the anesthetic solution. In addition, the baricity (a physical characteristic) of the local anesthetic, defined as the ratio between the density of the local anesthetic solution and the density of the CSF, will also determine the distribution: hyperbaric solutions move with gravity, effecting the greatest anesthetic results in the dependent areas; isobaric solutions will remain at the level of injection; and hypobaric solutions rise, effecting the greatest anesthetic results in the nondependent areas [9].

Choice of agents include:

Drug	Duration (min)	Dose (mg)
Lidocaine 5 %	60–75	50–70
Tetracaine 1 %	90–120	6–14
Prilocaine 2 %	100–130	40–60
Bupivacaine 0.75 %	120–150	10–14
Hyperbaric bupivacaine 0.5 %	120–150	10–15
Levobupivacaine 0.5 %	130–170	10–15
Ropivacaine 0.5 %	140–200	15–20

Opioids, such as fentanyl or intrathecal morphine, may also be administered with or without the local anesthetic. When used in combination with a local anesthetic, their ability to produce intense analgesia for long durations makes them ideal for postoperative pain management. Overall duration of the SAB is dependent on many factors, such as tissue uptake, vascular absorption, perfusion at the site of action, use of a co-administered vasoconstrictor, and factors that affect the spread of the local anesthetic, as mentioned earlier [10].

2.2.3   Intraoperative Side Effects of Spinal Anesthesia

Cardiovascular and respiratory complications can occur secondary to SAB. The most frequently occurring complication is hypotension, secondary to multifactorial reasons including decreased vascular resistance and diminished CO, preexisting hypovolemia or in those patients who have baseline systolic blood pressures typically below 120 mmHg. Hypotension may also occur due to a sensory level blockade above T4 and/or patients intraoperative position.

There are also multifactorial reasons for bradycardia to manifest, indirectly causing a hypotensive response, such as unopposed vagal tone from a high sympathectomy or a blockade reaching the level of the cardio accelerators (T1–T4).

In addition to hypotension and/or bradycardia, an inadvertent vascular injection of local anesthetic, or a combination of a sympathectomy combined with oversedation, can lead to ventricular arrhythmias which may eventually lead to cardiac arrest.

In the event that the local anesthetic reaches the level of the cervical spinal cord and brain stem, a total spinal is produced. Manifestations of a total spinal include severe hypotension and bradycardia, also leading to cardiac arrest. Other signs and symptoms include upper extremity weakness and loss of consciousness.

Side effects related to a compromised state of ventilation can be associated with the combination of the subarachnoid block and narcotics used to assist in sedation or in the addition of intrathecal opioids. In the event of a high blockade and/or a total spinal, intercostal muscle paralysis will lead to dyspnea and the inability to cough, causing intraoperative hypoxia.

In addition to these cardiovascular and pulmonary complications, the patient may also exhibit nausea and/or vomiting due to the unopposed vagal tone and/or the hypotension produced that will, in turn, decrease cerebral blood flow, effecting the chemotactic trigger zone.

2.2.4   Postoperative Side Effects of Spinal Anesthesia

Another potential side effect of SAB is urinary retention [11]. The SAB abolishes the sensation of urgency to void and also produces a total motor blockade of the bladders' detrusor muscle, eliminating its ability to contract. This will result in postoperative retention, which will persist based upon the duration of the sensory block above the S2 and S3 sacral segments.

Post-dural puncture headache (PDPH) occurs when CSF leaks transdurally through the puncture hole created by the spinal needle, resulting in the brain shifting lower within the cranium, which causes traction on the meninges and pain-sensitive intracranial nerves. Therefore, the choices of spinal needle, in addition to the degree of provider experience, are determining factors in the likelihood of PDPH occurrence. PDPH can occur up to 5 days post-puncture, depending on the patients' intravascular volume status and their time to upright position and ambulation. Symptoms can range from mild to severe, including intense headaches (specifically related to a change in posture to erect or semierect), diplopia, tinnitus, and nausea. Management is typically and initially conservative, including bed rest, analgesics, and proper hydration. If the symptoms do not subside, the patient can receive caffeine, either orally or by intravenous route. When symptoms persist, an epidural injection of saline, or an autologous epidural blood patch, can be administered [12].

2.3 Anesthetic Assistance for Bladder Injection of Botulinum Toxin in Patients with Spinal Cord Injury (for Treatment of Overactive Bladder)

The treatment of overactive bladder, secondary to neurogenic or idiopathic origins, has traditionally been managed by pharmacologic intervention with antimuscarinic agents [13]. Because of their lack of uroselectivity, these agents have accompanying systemic side effects that limit their usefulness. An effective alternative for the treatment of overactive bladder is the intradetrusor muscle injection of onabotulinum toxin A, a naturally occurring neurotoxin that inhibits the presynaptic release of acetylcholine, causing skeletal muscle paralysis. The toxin can be administered via a flexible or rigid cystoscope [14]. Anesthetic management can include a local anesthetic (lidocaine 2% liquid and viscous) administered by the urologist, conscious sedation for more anxious patients, and general anesthesia for extremely anxious or sensitive patients and for neurogenic patients who are at high risk for autonomic dysreflexia. When general anesthesia is contraindicated, SAB with a local anesthetic can be used.

References

1. Smith I. Anesthesia for laparoscopy with emphasis on outpatient laparoscopy. Anesthesiol Clin North America. 2007;19:21–41.
2. Cunningham A. Anesthetic implications of laparoscopic surgery. Yale J Biol Med. 1998;71:551–78.
3. Barker L. Positioning on the operating table. Updat Anaesth. 2002;15:2.
4. Gerges FJ, Kanazi G, Jabbour-khoury S. Anesthesia for laparoscopy: a review. J Clin Anesth. 2006;18:67–78.
5. Bernards CM, Hostetter LS. Epidural and spinal anesthesia. In: Barash PG et al., editors. Clinical anesthesia. 7th ed. Philadelphia: Lippincott, Williams & Wilkins; 2013. p. 905–36.

6. Fettes P, Jansson J, Wildsmith J. Failed spinal anaesthesia: mechanisms, management, and prevention. Br J Anaesth. 2009;102(6):739–48.
7. Guyton AC, Hall JE. Hemostasis and blood coagulation. In: Textbook of medical physiology. 13th ed. Philadelphia: W.B. Saunders; 2015. p. 483–93
8. Kleinman W. Spinal, epidural, and caudal blocks. In: Butterworth JF, Mackey DC, Wasnick JD, editors. Morgan & Mikhail's clinical anesthesiology. 5th ed. New York: McGraw-Hill; 2013. p. 937–74.
9. Chumsang L, Thongmee S. Levobupivacaine and bupivacaine in spinal anesthesia for transurethral endoscopic surgery. J Med Assoc Thai. 2006;89(8):1133–9.
10. Nagelhout JJ, Plaus KL. Local anesthetics. In: Nurse anesthesia. 5th ed. St. Louise: Elsevier Saunders; 2014. p. 125–44
11. Baldini G, Bagry H, Aprikian A, Carli F, Phil M. Postoperative urinary retention. Anesthesiology. 2009;110:1139–57.
12. Ghaleb A, Khorasani A, Mangar D. Post-dural puncture headache. Int J Gen Med. 2012;5:45–51.
13. Shergill IS, Arya M, Hamid R, Khastgir J, Patel HRH, Shah PJR. The importance of autonomic dysreflexia to the urologist. Br J Urol Int. 2003;93:923–6.
14. Nitti VW. Botulinum toxin for the treatment of idiopathic and neurogenic overactive bladder: state of the art. Rev Urol. 2006;8(4):198–208.

Preserving Continence during Laparoscopic (LRP) or Robot-Assisted Radical Prostatectomy (RARP)

3

Aurel Messas and Youness Ahallal

3.1 Introduction

Prostate cancer (PC) is currently being detected at an earlier clinical stage and smaller volume than 20 years ago, as a result of prostate-specific antigen (PSA) screening [1]. PSA screening has also resulted in earlier diagnosis and lower PC mortality as more and more patients present with organ-confined disease [2]. Thus, an increasing number of radical prostatectomy (RP) procedures have been performed over the years [3]. RP featured a high rate of complications and sequelae including blood loss, postoperative urinary incontinence, and erectile dysfunction. Postoperative urinary incontinence has been shown to be bothersome and has a relevant negative effect on the patient satisfaction and health-related quality of life (QoL) [4]. Nevertheless, the improvements in the knowledge of anatomy of the neurovascular bundles, the puboprostatic ligament, the posterior rhabdosphincter, the urinary sphincter, and the dorsal venous complex have led to an extraordinary improvement of the surgical technique and to the standardization of the retropubic RP [4–6]. Since Walsh's contribution, many authors have shared important updates in order to optimize the surgical technique, with the purpose of reducing RP-related urinary incontinence [7].

Sixteen years ago, some authors started using the laparoscopic approach aiming to minimize damages to the anatomic structure in order to assure the urinary continence [8]. In high-volume centers, laparoscopic radical prostatectomy (LRP) is associated with a 12-month urinary continence recovery up to 95 %, which is similar to the outcomes of the open RP (ORP) [9].

A. Messas (✉)
Urologic Surgery, Max Fourestier Hospital, Nanterre, France
e-mail: aurelmessas@gmail.com

Y. Ahallal
Department of Urology, Clinique de l'Alma, Paris, France

© Springer International Publishing Switzerland 2016
A. Carbone et al. (eds.), *Functional Urologic Surgery in Neurogenic and Oncologic Diseases*, Urodynamics, Neurourology and Pelvic Floor Dysfunctions, DOI 10.1007/978-3-319-29191-8_3

Robotic technology combining three-dimensional vision, optical magnification, and instruments with 7 degrees of freedom allows surgeons to perform meticulous, precise, and steady movements with a better preservation of the anatomical structures involved in urinary continence. The 12-month urinary recovery after robotic-assisted radical prostatectomy (RARP) in high-volume centers ranged from 84 to 97 % [9].

Authors evaluated invasiveness and tissue damage after open RP (ORP) and minimally invasive radical prostatectomy (MIRP). Four markers of acute-phase response (interleukin-6, interleukin-10, C-reactive protein, serum amyloid A) were evaluated before and after the procedure. They failed to show any statistically significant difference between the two approaches [10]. In contrast, Mikaye et al. reported a retrospective study evaluating tissue damage after open and laparoscopic procedures; they showed that the tissue damage markers were significantly lower in those patients treated laparoscopically [11].

Fracalanza et al. demonstrated in a single, nonrandomized, prospective trial that the tissue damage was significantly lower after RARP [12]. No paper evaluated the difference in tissue trauma determined by LRP and RARP so far.

3.2   Factors Influencing Continence after Laparoscopic or Robotic Prostatectomy

(a) Preoperative patient characteristics

Preoperative patient characteristics and very likely surgeon experience are the main predictive factors of continence recovery after MIRP [13–15]. Obesity and prostate volume could affect the probability of recovering urinary continence after RARP [13, 14]. Patient age, comorbidities, severity of lower urinary tract symptoms, and preoperative erectile dysfunction are significant predictors of urinary incontinence after MIRP [16, 17].

(b) Surgeon experience

Controversy surrounds the issue of the impact of surgeon experience and learning curve on the continence recovery after RARP. Two major prospective trials demonstrated a significant increase of the continence rate after a 500 cases experience [15, 18]. Likewise, excellent results were also reported by many authors including less than 500 cases [17, 19, 20].

(c) Surgical technique

– *Posterior musculofascial reconstruction with or without anterior reconstruction*

The most investigated aspect of the reconstructive steps of the MIRP is the impact of posterior and/or anterior reconstruction on early urinary continence recovery. At the beginning of the posterior reconstruction experience, two interrupted 3-0 Vicryl stitches were used to tie the cut end of the Denonvilliers' fascia to the rhabdosphincter/median fibrous raphe on either side of the midline. This reconstructed plane was fixed to the posterior bladder wall, 2 cm behind the bladder neck [4]. This maneuver aims at restoring the length of the urethrosphincteric complex, preventing its retraction, and reducing the tension on the vesicourethral anastomosis. It may also provide a posterior wedge to the urethrosphincteric complex to help its effective contraction. Gautam et al. did not find conclusive results in terms of early urinary continence recovery mainly because of the absence of a uniform surgical technique, continence definitions, and methods used in the few analyzed studies comparing posterior reconstruction with the standard technique [21]. However, in that article, some clinical series in which the posterior reconstruction was associated with an anterior restoration of the pelvis were included as well [22, 23].

In a prospective comparative study, Woo et al. reported a mean time to reach continence that was statistically significantly shorter in patients who underwent the posterior reconstruction [24]. In a nonrandomized prospective study, Coelho et al. evaluated the influence of a modified posterior reconstruction on urinary continence recovery 1 month after surgery [25]. 330 patients receiving a standard procedure had lower continence rates at 1 and 4 weeks after MIRP when compared to 473 patients having posterior reconstruction. Data at a longer follow-up showed overlapping results between the two techniques [25]. In a meta-analysis of studies reporting urinary continence recovery after RARP, cumulative data showed a small advantage in favor of posterior reconstruction 1 month after surgery [26]. On the other hand, cumulative analyses evaluating the effect of posterior reconstruction at 3 months and 6 months after RARP showed overlapping results between the two groups.

Globally, there is evidence showing a small advantage favoring posterior reconstruction over the standard technique 1 month after surgery. This observation is not confirmed at a longer follow-up raising questions about the real clinical benefit of this difference. Even though the positive impact of posterior reconstruction is lower than that initially assumed, the technique is simple, quick, and reproducible and could support delicate anastomosis.

Different anterior reconstruction techniques have been described. The most frequently used technique was reported by Steiner who showed the ventral fixation of the rhabdosphincter involving the puboprostatic ligaments bilaterally and comprising a median suspensory system of the pubic arch [27].

In 2008, Tewari et al. described the total reconstruction of the vesicourethral junction technique combining the posterior reconstruction to the reattachment of the pubic arch to the bladder neck after completion of the anastomosis [23], and in the same year, Menon et al. described the double-layer urethrovesical anastomosis [22]. In 2009, Patel described the anterior reconstruction using the periurethral suspension stitch [28]. This technique was associated with significantly better urinary continence recovery at 1 month and 3 months when compared to the standard technique.

There is globally a small advantage in favor of total reconstruction in improving the early continence after MIRP. No differences were noted after a longer follow-up. The total reconstruction of the rhabdosphincter seems to offer some advantages to improve urinary continence recovery.

– *Transperitoneal and extraperitoneal approach*

Chung et al. compared the urinary continence after transperitoneal and extraperitoneal RARP. One hundred five and 155 patients had transperitoneal and extraperitoneal RARP, respectively.

Postoperative potency and continence rates were similar between the groups. The study showed overlapping results in terms of 3-, 6-, and 12-month urinary continence recovery after both approaches; however, the extraperitoneal group had a faster recovery of continence compared with the transperitoneal group [29].

– *Bladder neck preservation*

Bladder neck preservation significantly improved the continence recovery rates 3 months and 1 year after RARP in comparison with bladder neck resection and reconstruction. Such a difference was not confirmed 2 years after the procedure [30]. In a prospective comparative study, Finley et al. reported significantly better early urinary continence rates in patients who performed a hypothermic nerve-sparing dissection using cold irrigation and an endorectal cooling balloon cycled with 48-C saline in comparison with those receiving a standard procedure [16].

– *Dorsal venous complex (DVC) management*

In a prospective nonrandomized comparative study, Lei et al. showed significantly better 6-month urinary continence rates in patients who underwent an athermal DVC division followed by selective suture ligation prior to anastomosis when compared to those receiving suture ligation before athermal DVC division. This advantage was not present at a longer follow-up [30].

– *Use of barbed suture*

In a randomized controlled trial, Sammon et al. compared barbed versus standard monofilament suture for urethrovesical anastomosis; he reported no difference in urinary continence recovery at 1-month follow-up [31].

The use of barbed suture was recently proposed with the aim of reducing the time needed to perform the reconstructive steps of the RARP procedure. The study published by Sammon et al. in 2011 showed that the use of barbed monofilament suture was associated with overlapping urinary continence recovery in comparison with the standard monofilament [31].

3.3 Comparing Open, Robotic, and Laparoscopic Radical Prostatectomy

The most critical issue in evaluating the impact of surgeon experience on the surgery outcomes is the impossibility of controlling for surgical skills and individual surgeon factors in building clinical trials. Similarly to open and laparoscopic surgeons, robotic ones do not all have the same level of surgical skills, regardless of their experience. Thus, the learning curve is variable and depends on individual factors; it's therefore difficult to generalize and gain a representative picture.

In most comparative studies, ORP was performed by many surgeons with varying levels of expertise. On the contrary, MIRP was usually performed by a small number of highly experienced urologists.

Many papers provided data on urinary continence recovery after ORP or LRP. Considering the fact that those studies included LRP patients at the initial laparoscopy experience (knowing the slow learning curve associated with the LRP learning), the continence recovery was better after ORP [32]. Considering experience after the learning curve of LRP, the best evidence was in the paper from Touijer et al. who showed a statistically significant difference in favor of ORP; patients undergoing LRP had a higher risk of being incontinent. Patients who underwent LRP were less likely to become continent than those treated with retropubic ORP (HR 0.56 for laparoscopic vs. open radical prostatectomy) [33]. However, the cumulative analysis reported by Ficarra et al. showed the continence rates after ORP or LRP to be similar even when the evaluation was limited to only prospective studies [26].

Concerning the comparison between ORP and RARP, good evidence is provided by the paper from Tewari et al., who showed that the median time to continence was significantly shorter after RARP [34]. Kim et al. reported overlapping results between the two techniques. However, when the authors excluded the first 132 cases performed from the analysis, the median time to continence in RARP patients was significantly lower when compared to that reported in the ORP patients [35].

Ficarra et al. included five studies in the cumulative analysis evaluating the 12-month urinary continence recovery after RARP or ORP [26]. The absolute risk of urinary incontinence was 11.3% after ORP (105 of 923 cases) and 7.5% after RARP (38 of 509 cases). Therefore, the absolute risk reduction was 3.8%. Authors showed a significant advantage favoring RARP in the urinary continence recovery; the cumulative analysis showed a statistically significant advantage in favor of RARP (OR, 1.53; 95% CI, 1.04–2.25; $p = 0.03$) [26].

The only study comparing urinary continence after LRP and RARP failed to show any difference in the 6-month postoperative continence rates [36].

Data from the available comparative studies suggested that advantage in terms of urinary continence and erectile function might be present in patients having RARP compared with those having ORP. Specifically, quicker recovery of continence and potency were shown for patients having RARP compared with those undergoing ORP [35], while no significant differences were found in both outcomes comparing RARP with LRP [34, 36].

Ficarra et al. included five studies in the cumulative analysis evaluating the 12-month urinary continence recovery after RARP or LRP [26]. The absolute risk of urinary incontinence was 9.6% after LRP (29 of 302 cases) and 5% after RARP (22 of 436 cases). Therefore, the absolute risk reduction was 4.6%, and patients treated with LRP were more likely to be incontinent compared to those treated robotically. The cumulative analysis showed a statistically significant advantage in favor of RARP.

The same authors demonstrated, for the first time, significant advantages for RARP in comparison with ORP in terms of 12-month urinary continence rates.

These results do not seem to be influenced by data coming from referral high-volume centers.

In 2009, Hu et al. reported significantly higher urinary incontinence rates after MIRP in comparison with ORP. However, no differences were reported in the number of procedures performed to treat that complication [37].

The same conclusions were drawn in a Surveillance, Epidemiology, and End Results (SEER) registry cohort of patients treated between 2002 and 2005. Therefore, the comparison between the different approaches was significantly limited by the learning curve of the MIRP surgeons. Later, Barry et al. published a new population-based study analyzing 685 patients (≥65 years old) who were treated with RARP or ORP during 2008. A cross-sectional analysis performed 14 months after surgery using a non-validated questionnaire showed similar results between RARP and ORP when it comes to urinary continence bother [38].

Nevertheless, many limitations have to be acknowledged in such a study: several MIRP surgeons were still probably in their learning curve, no baseline urinary function was reported, all patients were ≥65 years of age, no information concerning surgical techniques was reported, and only a non-validated questionnaire evaluating bother was used [38].

3.4   Limitations

We have to acknowledge upfront many limitations from a methodological point of view, limitations concerning the quality of the available studies, the definition of continence from one study to another, and the methods used for data collection. Regarding the continence definition, the most relevant confounding factor was the acceptance of the safety pad. Interestingly, Ficarra et al. proposed a standardized classification distinguishing patients not using pads (C0) from those using a safety pad (C1) or multiple pads (C2). This classification should be strongly considered in future studies in order to perform adequate comparative analyses [39].

References

1. Descazeaud A, et al. Can pT0 stage of prostate cancer be predicted before radical prostatectomy? Eur Urol. 2006;50(6):1248–52; discussion 1253.
2. Jemal A, et al. Cancer statistics, 2009. CA Cancer J Clin. 2009;59(4):225–49.
3. Schroder FH, et al. Early detection of prostate cancer in 2007. Part 1: PSA and PSA kinetics. Eur Urol. 2008;53(3):468–77.
4. Rocco F, et al. Restoration of posterior aspect of rhabdosphincter shortens continence time after radical retropubic prostatectomy. J Urol. 2006;175(6):2201–6.
5. Walsh PC, Donker PJ. Impotence following radical prostatectomy: insight into etiology and prevention. J Urol. 1982;128(3):492–7.
6. Myers RP, Goellner JR, Cahill DR. Prostate shape, external striated urethral sphincter and radical prostatectomy: the apical dissection. J Urol. 1987;138(3):543–50.
7. Steiner MS, Morton RA, Walsh PC. Impact of anatomical radical prostatectomy on urinary continence. J Urol. 1991;145(3):512–4; discussion 514–5.

8. Guillonneau B, et al. Laparoscopic radical prostatectomy: technical and early oncological assessment of 40 operations. Eur Urol. 1999;36(1):14–20.
9. Ficarra V, et al. Retropubic, laparoscopic, and robot-assisted radical prostatectomy: a systematic review and cumulative analysis of comparative studies. Eur Urol. 2009;55(5):1037–63.
10. Jurczok A, et al. Prospective non-randomized evaluation of four mediators of the systemic response after extraperitoneal laparoscopic and open retropubic radical prostatectomy. BJU Int. 2007;99(6):1461–6.
11. Miyake H, et al. Comparison of surgical stress between laparoscopy and open surgery in the field of urology by measurement of humoral mediators. Int J Urol. 2002;9(6):329–33.
12. Fracalanza S, et al. Is robotically assisted laparoscopic radical prostatectomy less invasive than retropubic radical prostatectomy? Results from a prospective, unrandomized, comparative study. BJU Int. 2008;101(9):1145–9.
13. Link BA, et al. The impact of prostate gland weight in robot assisted laparoscopic radical prostatectomy. J Urol. 2008;180(3):928–32.
14. Wiltz AL, et al. Robotic radical prostatectomy in overweight and obese patients: oncological and validated-functional outcomes. Urology. 2009;73(2):316–22.
15. Zorn KC, et al. Continued improvement of perioperative, pathological and continence outcomes during 700 robot-assisted radical prostatectomies. Can J Urol. 2009;16(4):4742–9; discussion 4749.
16. Finley DS, et al. Hypothermic robotic radical prostatectomy: impact on continence. J Endourol. 2009;23(9):1443–50.
17. Novara G, et al. Evaluating urinary continence and preoperative predictors of urinary continence after robot assisted laparoscopic radical prostatectomy. J Urol. 2010;184(3):1028–33.
18. Samadi DB, et al. Improvements in robot-assisted prostatectomy: the effect of surgeon experience and technical changes on oncologic and functional outcomes. J Endourol. 2010;24(7):1105–10.
19. Murphy DG, et al. Operative details and oncological and functional outcome of robotic-assisted laparoscopic radical prostatectomy: 400 cases with a minimum of 12 months follow-up. Eur Urol. 2009;55(6):1358–66.
20. Martin AD, et al. Incontinence after radical prostatectomy: a patient centered analysis and implications for preoperative counseling. J Urol. 2011;186(1):204–8.
21. Gautam G, et al. Posterior rhabdosphincter reconstruction during robot-assisted radical prostatectomy: critical analysis of techniques and outcomes. Urology. 2010;76(3):734–41.
22. Menon M, et al. Assessment of early continence after reconstruction of the periprostatic tissues in patients undergoing computer assisted (robotic) prostatectomy: results of a 2 group parallel randomized controlled trial. J Urol. 2008;180(3):1018–23.
23. Tewari A, et al. Total reconstruction of the vesico-urethral junction. BJU Int. 2008;101(7):871–7.
24. Woo JR, et al. Impact of posterior rhabdosphincter reconstruction during robot-assisted radical prostatectomy: retrospective analysis of time to continence. J Endourol. 2009;23(12):1995–9.
25. Coelho RF, et al. Influence of modified posterior reconstruction of the rhabdosphincter on early recovery of continence and anastomotic leakage rates after robot-assisted radical prostatectomy. Eur Urol. 2011;59(1):72–80.
26. Ficarra V, et al. Systematic review and meta-analysis of studies reporting urinary continence recovery after robot-assisted radical prostatectomy. Eur Urol. 2012;62(3):405–17.
27. Steiner MS. The puboprostatic ligament and the male urethral suspensory mechanism: an anatomic study. Urology. 1994;44(4):530–4.
28. Patel VR, et al. Periurethral suspension stitch during robot-assisted laparoscopic radical prostatectomy: description of the technique and continence outcomes. Eur Urol. 2009;56(3):472–8.
29. Chung JS, et al. Comparison of oncological results, functional outcomes, and complications for transperitoneal versus extraperitoneal robot-assisted radical prostatectomy: a single surgeon's experience. J Endourol. 2011;25(5):787–92.
30. Lei Y, et al. Athermal division and selective suture ligation of the dorsal vein complex during robot-assisted laparoscopic radical prostatectomy: description of technique and outcomes. Eur Urol. 2011;59(2):235–43.

31. Sammon J, et al. Anastomosis during robot-assisted radical prostatectomy: randomized controlled trial comparing barbed and standard monofilament suture. Urology. 2011;78(3):572–9.
32. Krane LS, et al. Posterior support for urethrovesical anastomosis in robotic radical prostatectomy: single surgeon analysis. Can J Urol. 2009;16(5):4836–40.
33. Touijer K, et al. Comprehensive prospective comparative analysis of outcomes between open and laparoscopic radical prostatectomy conducted in 2003 to 2005. J Urol. 2008;179(5):1811–7; discussion 1817.
34. Tewari A, et al. A prospective comparison of radical retropubic and robot-assisted prostatectomy: experience in one institution. BJU Int. 2003;92(3):205–10.
35. Kim SC, et al. Factors determining functional outcomes after radical prostatectomy: robot-assisted versus retropubic. Eur Urol. 2011;60(3):413–9.
36. Joseph JV, et al. Robot-assisted vs pure laparoscopic radical prostatectomy: are there any differences? BJU Int. 2005;96(1):39–42.
37. Hu JC, et al. Comparative effectiveness of minimally invasive vs open radical prostatectomy. JAMA. 2009;302(14):1557–64.
38. Barry MJ, et al. Adverse effects of robotic-assisted laparoscopic versus open retropubic radical prostatectomy among a nationwide random sample of medicare-age men. J Clin Oncol. 2012;30(5):513–8.
39. Ficarra V, et al. Systematic review of methods for reporting combined outcomes after radical prostatectomy and proposal of a novel system: the survival, continence, and potency (SCP) classification. Eur Urol. 2012;61(3):541–8.

Selecting Patients for Continent or Incontinent, Heterotopic or Orthotopic Diversion

4

Antonio Carbone and Andrea Fuschi

Radical cystectomy (RC) and urinary diversions (UDs) are difficult procedures in urology, especially when RC is performed by mini-invasive technique (laparoscopic/robotic) and UDs are tailored intracorporeally. However, RC remains the best treatment option for *muscle-invasive bladder cancer* (MIBC) or high-risk *non-invasive bladder cancer* (NIBC) [1, 2]. Different UD procedures have their own indications and may present specific problems. In experienced hands and high-volume centers with rigorous standardized preoperative selection and systematic long-term follow-up, major complications can be avoided and excellent long-term results can be achieved.

Primary goals in selecting a UD are to provide the lowest rate of perioperative complications and the highest postoperative health-related quality of life (HRQoL). Thus, either a timely start or completion of chemotherapy and the therapeutic goals is more likely to be reached.

For this reason, a number of factors should be considered while counseling each patient to choose the best diversion. However, patients must be informed that intraoperative findings may dictate a change in the planned UD (e.g., positive urethral margin precluding orthotopic diversion). In fact, even when an orthotopic neobladder is planned, all patients should have a stoma site marked preoperatively by an enterostomal therapist in the event that orthotopic diversion becomes unfeasible.

The most important factors to be considered can be divided in two categories: *clinicopathological features of cancer* and *patient's individual features*.

A. Carbone (✉) • A. Fuschi
Urology Unit, Department of Medico-Surgical Sciences and Biotechnologies,
Sapienza University of Rome, Polo Pontino, Latina, Italy
e-mail: antonio.carbone@uniroma1.it

© Springer International Publishing Switzerland 2016
A. Carbone et al. (eds.), *Functional Urologic Surgery in Neurogenic and Oncologic Diseases*, Urodynamics, Neurourology and Pelvic Floor Dysfunctions, DOI 10.1007/978-3-319-29191-8_4

4.1   Clinicopathological Features

According to the European Association of Urology (EAU) Guidelines, RC is rec-ommended for patients with MIBC T2-T4a, N0-Nx, and M0 [3]. Other indications include high-risk recurrent superficial tumors (T1G3) or bacillus Calmette-Guerin (BCG)-resistant carcinoma in situ (Tis). Tumor stage can strongly influence the decision-making about continent or incontinent urinary diversion; in fact, even in case of positive lymph nodes, when the metastasis is in a single node of the true pelvis (N1), an orthotopic neobladder can still be considered [4]. Otherwise, the tumor involvement of the prostatic urethra in males and of the bladder neck in females should exclude an orthotopic UD.

4.1.1   Locally Advanced Tumor Stage

In the routine practice, for many urologists, a locally extensive disease may be a contraindication to perform an orthotopic diversion. This is due to two principal factors:

1. Possible local recurrence in the neobladder
2. Concern that these patients may shortly be affected by distant recurrence, doomed to a shortened life expectancy

Radical cystectomy with bilateral pelvic-iliac lymphadenectomy (LND) pro-vides excellent local (pelvic) control of invasive bladder cancer. In the series by Stein et al. (2001), in 1,054 patients who underwent RC for bladder cancer with a median follow-up of more than 10 years, an overall local pelvic recurrence rate of 7 % was observed [5]. These results suggest that, even for patients suffering from locally advanced or positive lymph node disease, local recurrence is relatively infre-quent and should not necessarily preclude any form of UDs. Approximately 50 % of patients with advanced tumor extension and 30 % of the patients with positive lymph node disease were still alive without evidence of cancer at 5 years of follow-up [5]. The EAU guidelines for muscle-invasive and metastatic bladder cancer [6] recommend RC as the standard treatment for localized MIBC in most Western countries [3, 5]. Nevertheless, recent interest in patients' quality of life (QoL) has promoted the trend toward bladder-preserving treatment modalities, such as radio-and/or chemotherapy. Age and performance status (PS) should influence the choice of primary therapy, as well as patients' own preference about the type of UD. Cystectomy should then be reserved to younger subjects without concomitant diseases and a good PS. In a multivariate analysis, Miller DC et al. confirmed the importance to assess the overall health status before recommending and proceeding with surgery [7]. This analysis found an association between comorbidity and adverse pathological or survival outcomes following RC [7]. Performance status and comorbidity have a different impact on treatment outcomes and must be inde-pendently evaluated [8].

4.1.2   Urethral Tumor Involvement in Man

Urothelial carcinoma in the urethral stump is one of the most important contraindications for orthotopic UD due to the risk of a cancer recurrence involving neobladder-urethral anastomosis. In fact the involvement of prostatic urethra is associated with a higher risk for urethral tumor recurrence after RC. One of the first studies reporting this statement was published in 1956 [9], and other authors confirmed this finding later [10–15]. The overall probability of urethral recurrence was estimated to be approximately 7 % at 5 years and 9 % at 10 years. Recurrences were observed at a median of 2 years after RC (range 0.2–13 years). The risk at 5 years was only 5 % in patients with prostate tumor involvement compared with 11 % for those without it [16]. Stenzl et al., in a large pooled analysis of 25 case series involving 3,165 patients undergoing cystectomy for bladder cancer, reported 8.1 % of anterior urethral tumor recurrences. This risk was related to the primary bladder cancer characteristics, including multifocality or tumor involvement of the trigone, bladder neck, prostate, upper urinary tract, and Tis in the bladder [17, 18]. The degree of prostatic involvement is of utmost importance to predict the risk of subsequent urethral recurrence. We should, thus, consider three different possible pathological scenarios:

(a) Urethral mucosa involvement (including Tis)
(b) Ductal involvement with Tis
(c) Prostatic stromal invasion

Only urethral mucosa involvement appears to be not associated with increased recurrence. Patients presenting prostatic ductal and prostatic stromal involvement developed 25 % and 64 % of urethral recurrence, respectively [12]. Levinson et al. in 1990 reported similar rates of recurrence while Hassan and colleagues in 2004 reported a lower risk although based on a relatively short follow-up [13, 19].

All these studies confirm that prostatic stromal invasion is the single strongest pathological predictor of recurrence in the anterior urethra after RC for bladder cancer. Tis and tumor multifocality, on the other hand, do not appear to be associated with a significant risk for it [16].

There is some debate regarding the importance to identify prostatic urethral involvement preoperatively. At the time of transurethral resection (TURB) of the primary bladder tumor, it might be useful to take deep transurethral resection biopsies of the prostate, preferably at the 5- and 7-o'clock positions lateral to the verumontanum. This appears to be particularly important if the mucosa of the prostatic urethra looks suspicious or when primary tumor involves the bladder neck. Some authors have recommended these biopsies to be done routinely and have advocated repeating transurethral resection (TUR) before cystectomy in patients where this was omitted [20, 21]. Other authors disapproved this practice, stating that intraoperative frozen section analysis is more accurate in predicting urethral recurrence rather than any other preoperative assessment, including prostate biopsies [22, 23]. Moreover it is questionable whether the supplementary information garnered by a repeated TUR with prostatic urethral biopsy justifies the risk of additional anesthesia and the potential delay to definitive surgery. However, if an orthotopic UD is selected, the authors will depend, at the end, on the intraoperative frozen section of the urethral margin performed just under the verumontanum for the final decision. When there are positive lymph nodes, orthotopic neobladder can nevertheless be considered in the case of N1 involvement (metastasis in a single node in the true pelvis) but not for N2 or N3 tumors [24].

4.1.3   Urethral Tumor Involvement in Women

The concept of continent neobladder in men has led a number of investigators to evaluate the preservation of the urethra in women too.

The studies of Stein and Stenzl were critical to expand urethral-preserving cystectomy to women with urothelial carcinoma.

In the first study all female patients with an uninvolved bladder neck had also an uninvolved urethra [25]. Also the results of Stenzl confirm that the bladder neck involvement was the most significant risk factor for secondary urethral tumor in women [17]. In fact, approximately 50 % of patients with a bladder neck tumor had concomitant urethral involvement; moreover, increased grade of tumor, stage, and lymph node involvement were associated with the risk for urethral involvement, while the presence of Tis did not predict urethral spread. Another important risk factor for urethral recurrence in women is vaginal wall involvement that determines 50 % of urethral extension [25].

These studies both concluded that the urethra could be safely preserved in selected female patients submitted to RC provided that neither preoperative biopsy specimens of the bladder neck nor intraoperative frozen section specimens of the proximal urethra demonstrate any tumor or atypia [17]. The shorter length of the female urethra resulting in a smaller area of transitional cell mucosa appears to be the reason of a lower incidence of urethral tumors in women. In addition, the area *"at risk"* in the female urethra seems to decrease with increasing age being replaced by metaplastic squamous cells. In the sixth and seventh decades of life, when most bladder tumors occur, metaplastic squamous cell mucosa generally covers the entire urethra, the bladder neck, and even a portion of the trigone [26]. For this reason, also in women, Stein et al. suggest that preoperative biopsy of the bladder neck or urethra is not necessary, but the decision to preserve the urethra may rely upon the intraoperative frozen section to take the final decision for orthotopic UD [25, 27, 28]. As previously mentioned for men, in the case of N1 involvement (metastasis in a single node in the true pelvis), orthotopic neobladder can still be considered but not for N2 or N3 tumors [4, 24].

4.2   Patient's Individual Features

This issue includes the patient's general health and social status, age, QoL, presence of a functional urethra, renal function, previous pelvic radiotherapy, prostate surgery, bowel disease/resection, and manual dexterity. Another important point is the evaluation of the patient's personal preference in relation to the risk of incontinence, need of self-catheterization, and management of an external device. The patient and his or her relatives must have a realistic understanding of the pros and cons of each type of UD before the concluding decision. Most patients prefer to opt for an orthotopic reconstruction because it seems the most "natural"; during the counseling they need to be informed that problems can occur with any type of UD and an honest, informed discussion, carefully explaining the various options of UD, must be addressed.

4.2.1   Age

Among the authors there is consensus on the fact that age cannot be considered an absolute contraindication for RC and UDs because other elements must be considered first. Lance (2001), Clark (2005), and Sogni et al. (2008) reported the possible favorable outcome of continent UD in elderly patients that, although those treated by orthotopic technique may regain continence more slowly and have a higher rate of mild stress incontinence, they can achieve a good continence rate comparable to younger patients [29–32]. In these patients, the medical (renal, cardiac, pulmonary) comorbidities and other issues such as cognitive function and the possible patient's support by caregivers should be considered. Certainly in a frail, sedentary, elderly person, a conduit may be easier to be managed for a caregiver than an orthotopic UD with a higher risk of daily clean intermittent catheterization and/or incontinence. Hereafter, keeping in mind all these considerations, an elderly patient <80 years may certainly be considered a possible candidate for RC and UDs even if orthotopic.

4.2.2   Health-Related Quality of Life (HRQoL)

Another reason for selecting a UD is the preservation of a "normal" body image. Many reports have emphasized improvements in various specific aspects of HRQoL, e.g., body image, with these reconstructive techniques; few formal studies have documented an improvement in overall HRQoL. In literature, there is no any evidence of better HRQoL outcomes in patients undergoing orthotopic than other types of UD. For example, the Vanderbilt group analyzed RAND 36-Item Health Survey (SF-36) and Functional Assessment of Cancer Therapy-General (FACT-G) questionnaires from 29 pts with an ileal conduit compared with 42 pts with orthotopic UD [33]. Although they reported advantages in HRQoL for those receiving an orthotopic diversion, this cohort of patients had a younger average age, and this can be considered a bias. In addition, the Los Angeles (UCLA) group, by the University of California, produced a systematic overview of 15 published studies about HRQoL after RC and UD for bladder cancer [34] but none of them was randomized, except one prospective in its design.

More specific experiences in literature focus on the assessment of QoL in patients submitted to RC and orthotopic UD. Siracusano in 2014 developed a dedicated questionnaire, named "IONB-PRO" (IONB (ileal orthotopic neobladder)), and validated it performing a trial on 145 patients. The questionnaire showed a high level of internal consistency and reliability with an excellent discriminant validity. This tool may be used instead of not specific and generic questionnaires [35]. A subsequent Italian multicenter observational study based on this questionnaire involving 174 subjects from January 2010 to December 2013 showed that age, urinary incontinence, length of follow-up, and comorbidity status may influence postoperative HRQoL and should all be taken into account when counseling RC-IONB patients [36].

However there is no any worldwide consensus available to conclude that a better HRQoL is associated to any form of UD for the lack of long-term longitudinal studies using reliable measures and validated instrument.

4.2.3 Renal Function

Two concepts should be considered regarding the possibility that renal dysfunction may represent an important contraindication for continent neobladder reconstruction:

(a) Patients submitted to UD are likely exposed to complications (hydronephrosis, neobladder-ureteral reflux) which could increase the risk of kidney failure;

(b) Small-bowel mucosa, utilized for UD, may cause reabsorption of urinary electrolytes (urea, potassium, and bicarbonate) increasing the acid load that must be handled by the kidneys. Therefore, a compromised renal function may determine hyperchloremic metabolic acidosis, worsening dehydration, uremia, nausea, and bone loss.

Nowadays there is no a fixed level of acceptable renal function to choose different diversions. Obviously, an acute upper urinary tract obstruction, caused by an external compression (e.g., by the tumor) and resulting in a transient rise of creatinine, often improves after cystectomy. Generally a serum creatinine <1.7–2.2 mg/dL (150–200 μmol/L) or an estimated creatinine clearance >35–40 mL/min would be considered acceptable [3, 37]. However, decision must be made on any single case.

4.2.4 Obesity

Obesity is not a contraindication for this procedure. However, an increased BMI should be considered a specific risk factor both for surgical and anesthesiologic reasons due to several comorbidities associated with pathological condition (see Chap. 2). From a surgical point of view, the thickened bowel mesentery and the thick abdominal wall can make more difficult to perform an orthotopic diversion and also the creation of a stoma.

4.2.5   Manual Dexterity for Self-Catheterization

Hautmann et al. (2007) stated that 10–50 % of men and 30–50 % of women might need occasional or routine self-catheterization after UD [3]. Of course all patients receiving a continent pouch need clean intermittent catheterization (CIC) or other types of urinary collectors and, before surgery, have to be informed about this and extensively instructed regarding CIC management and the wide selection of devices on the market.

In patients suitable for an orthotopic neobladder, it is generally impossible to predict which patients will require CIC to achieve a complete emptying. Partial or complete urinary retention can occur early or years after the procedure. For this reason patients eligible for continent UDs, ortho- or heterotopic, should have a sufficient manual dexterity to do CIC and be informed, counseled, and trained about devices and methods for it. It seems an obvious statement but the surgeon must consider that, when a cutaneous stoma is needed, the side position of it is conditioned to the manual dexterity (right/left handed).

4.2.6   Previous Radiotherapy of the Pelvis

Scarring around the rabdomyosphincter area is increased after previous external beam radiation (EBRT) and brachytherapy for prostate cancer in male or cervical cancer in female, in comparison with EBRT for bladder or colon cancer. In case of brachytherapy, the site of seeds implant can influence this possible consequence. Therefore, in these patients cystoscopy is mandatory for any eventually preoperative evaluation to assess the integrity of the mucosa around the area of the sphincter when an orthotopic UD is planned. However, it cannot be possible to exactly predict the degree of radiation damage that will be found at surgery. Thus, a careful intraoperative tissue assessment of the urethra, ureters, and bowel must be performed to make a final decision about the feasibility of orthotopic UD [38]. These patients should always be counseled preoperatively that an orthotopic diversion might not be possible.

Stein et al. found that 8.5 % of 1,471 patients who needed RC for MIBC had received radiation therapy for previous pelvic malignancy (e.g., prostate cancer) and that this exposure caused a more difficult surgical procedure, compromising wound healing and postoperative outcomes [5]. Ahlering et al., in a retrospective matched analysis, compared 86 patients undergoing RC with cutaneous continent diversion of which 44 had a history of prior radiation and 42 who did not [39]. They found no significant difference between irradiated and not irradiated patients in terms of operative time, blood loss, transfusion rate, and wound or ureteral complications [39]. Gschwend et al. concluded that high-dose pelvic irradiation should not be a primary contraindication for orthotopic UD with segments of the small intestine, considering the duration of hospital stay, perioperative complications, and early functional results. The postoperative course in this group did not differ from that of a control group of non-irradiated patients [40]. Bochner et al. analyzed a total of 18 patients who had failed radiation treatment (total minimum dose, ≥60 Gy) for bladder or prostate cancer and had undergone orthotopic UD. They found similar operative and postoperative outcomes in irradiated and non-irradiated patients and suggested that the orthotopic UDs appear to be safe, effective procedures that provide a functional lower urinary tract in those patients in which definitive pelvic radiation therapy has failed [41, 42]. In conclusion, in eligible patients, orthotopic lower urinary tract reconstruction can be performed nevertheless previous pelvic irradiation. However, these are challenging procedures that clearly require technical expertise and well-equipped institution.

4.2.7 Previous Prostate Surgery or Bowel Preoperative Status

Previous abdominal or pelvic surgery (e.g., radical prostatectomy, RP) may also present challenges for the surgeon performing orthotopic UD, especially during the dissection around the proximal urethra or at the site of the prior vesicourethral anastomosis. Huang et al. in their experience with 1,900 cases found that the patients with a history of previous RP and a good postoperative continence had a fair chance of regaining good urinary control with the neobladder reconstruction after RC [43]. It should also be taken into consideration that in previous abdominal surgery, when multiple bowel resections have been done, the additional removal of 45–60 cm of the small bowel to create a complex UD can cause chronic diarrhea or even a "short bowel syndrome." In those patients an alternative UD to orthotopic neobladder can be indicated. Besides, even patients suffering from inflammatory bowel disease as ulcerative colitis, Crohn's disease, or diverticulosis may be better served by a bowel conduit [44].

4.3 Laparoscopic Radical Cystectomy and Intracorporeal Urinary Diversion: Patient Selection, Techniques, and Outcomes

4.3.1 Patient Selection

Radical cystectomy with pelvic lymph node dissection (PLND) and UD is the gold standard treatment for MIBC [5].

Making a decision about the most appropriate UD to be selected for a single patient has to be considered an important and not an easy detail. All the abovementioned clinicopathological and individual features of the patients have to be considered, but the final program should be decided in total agreement with the patient during a complete and exhaustive counseling.

In our institution according to the general health condition of the patients, the disease-specific condition, the expected free-disease survival, and the patient's expectation on postoperative QoL, we are used to suggest these diversions from the technically easier to the most difficult:

Uretero – cutaneostomy → uretero – ileo – cutaneostomy →
U – shaped orthotopic neobladder → VIP – shaped orthotopic neobladder →
Hemi – Koch pouch continent diversion

From 2012 in our institution both cystectomy and diversions are performed by a fully intracorporeal laparoscopic approach similarly to the other major oncologic routine procedures for prostate and kidney cancers (see Graphs 4.1 and 4.2) [45].

Minimally invasive surgical approaches for cystectomy have been described since 1992, when laparoscopic radical cystectomy (LRC) was first reported [46, 47] to reduce morbidity and decrease the hospital stay. High costs, technical difficulties,

Graph 4.1 Rate between laparoscopic and open procedure for major surgery at Urology Unit – "La Sapienza" University – Polo Pontino

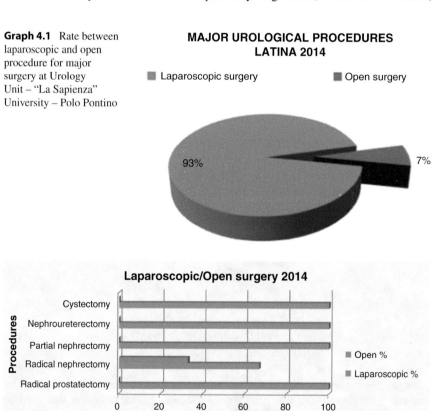

Graph 4.2 Different rates between laparoscopic and open procedure for major surgery divided for surgical technique/diseases at Urology Unit – "La Sapienza" University – Polo Pontino

tough learning curve, and exhausting operative time hampered the immediate widespread adoption of these techniques [48], but now its broader use is being facilitated by the development of new dissection and hemostatic devices that simplify some surgical steps. This also assured better oncologic and functional outcomes [49].

The intracorporeal reconstruction of an orthotopic neobladder was described in 2000 [50]. Since then, expertise with laparoscopic surgery has increased, with a greater interest in this procedure and the consequent report of different reconstructive options. LRC and robot-assisted RC (RARC) with intracorporeal UD reconstruction have been demonstrated to be feasible, safe, and capable of providing many operative and functional advantages [51, 52].

In our institute the inclusion criteria for LRC + orthotopic UDs included:

(a) MIBC (T2–4a), N0–Nx, and M0
(b) High-risk or recurrent non-muscle-invasive tumors or multifocal T1G3
(c) T1G3 with concomitant carcinoma in situ (CIS)

Patients are not considered eligible for these procedures in case of:

(a) Refusal of LRC with orthotopic diversion
(d) Oncologic contraindication to LRC including urethral tumor involvement or distant metastases
(e) General contraindication to laparoscopy, as for the American Society of Anaesthesiologists (ASA) score >3, severe heart and/or respiratory failure
(f) Specific contraindications to neobladder diversion as the presence of a urethral stricture, previous extensive abdominal surgery, or severely insufficient renal function

We consider relative contraindications for LRC an age >75 years and a body mass index (BMI) >30.

4.3.2 Techniques

With the patient placed in a supine, steep Trendelenburg position (20–25°), pneumoperitoneum (12 mmHg) is established. A five-port, fan-shaped, transperitoneal approach is used, according to the Hasson technique [53]. A standard bilateral pelvic lymphadenectomy is usually performed as the first step. The boundaries of standard PLND are the bifurcation of the common iliac artery, proximally; the genitofemoral nerve, laterally; the circumflex iliac vein and lymph node of Cloquet, distally; and the hypogastric vessels, posteriorly, including the obturator fossa. Extended PLND (in order to reach the aortic bifurcation) is performed in all cT3 cases and when computed tomography reveals a pelvic lymphadenopathy.

After PLND, the Douglas pouch is transversely incised, and the umbilical liga-ments and urachus are divided by a 5-mm radio-frequency device (Ligasure-Covidien, Boulder, CO, USA) allowing for entry into the Retzius space to mobilize the bladder. The ureters are isolated bilaterally, at the crossing with the iliac artery or with the deferens, and then clipped with a Hem-o-lok and transected with cold scissors, just outside the bladder; the distal margins of the ureters are also sent for frozen section biopsy. Deferens are transected bilaterally, and the seminal vesicles dissected and fixed to the bladder using a 5-mm Hem-o-lok (Teleflex Medical, Research Triangle Park, NC, USA). The Denonvilliers' fascia is then incised, and the fatty space between the rectum and the prostate is developed. Endopelvic fascia is incised bilaterally, and the lateral pedicles of the bladder and prostate are divided using Hem-o-lok clips, cold scissors, and bipolar forceps; to prevent thermal injury to the neurovascular bundles, the apex of the prostate, urethra, and rectourethral muscles are divided using scissors.

Puboprostatic ligaments and the dorsal vein complex are transected by radiofrequency.

In youngest patients, willing to preserve erectile function, the endopelvic fascia is not incised bilaterally from the beginning but the virtual space within the prostate and the neurovascular bundle is developed from the seminal vesicle and prostatic base to the apex by cold scissor, bipolar forceps and titanium clips using an intra-fascial or interfascial plane. Then the neurovascular bundle is lateralized and the endopelvic fascia incised bilaterally to spare at the best the anterior aspect of the Aphrodite veil; the puboprostatic ligaments and the dorsal vein complex are dis-sected by radiofrequency (Fig. 4.1a, b).

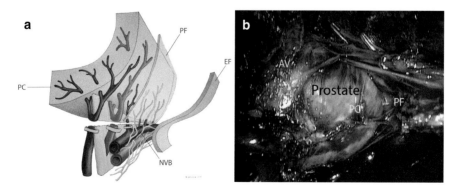

Fig. 4.1 (**a**) A schematic representation of visceral layer of the endopelvic fascia (*EF*) and of the prostatic fascia (*PF*). These two distinct fascias surround the prostatic capsule (*PC*). The virtual space within the prostate and the neurovascular bundles (*NVB*) is developed from the seminal vesicle and prostatic base to the apex without incising the endopelvic fascia bilaterally using an intrafascial or interfascial plane. (**b**) Intraoperative aspect of the posterolateral dissection of the prostate (see **a**). (*PF* prostatic fascia, *AV* Aphrodite veil, *PC* prostatic capsule)

4.3.2.1 U-Shaped Neobladder (U-n) Reconfiguration and Vescica Ileale Padovana Neobladder (VIP-n) Reconfiguration

For both reconfigurations, a 40-cm segment of the ileum, 20 cm from the ileocecal junction, is selected and transected. Ileoileal continuity is restored using Endo-GIA staplers (US Surgical, Norwalk, CT, USA).

For the U-n the selected ileal segment is detubularized, and a globular U-shaped ileal neobladder is tailored approximating the two afferent and efferent loops of the ileum and suturing them by two subsequent charges of Endo-GIA staplers [45].

For the VIP-n reconstruction, the afferent and efferent loops of the selected ileal segment are approximated in a U shape with a longer left arm. Two holes are then opened at the caudal third segment of the U-shaped ileal loop, and through them, the distal funnel of the VIP-n is created by a single charge of Endo-GIA stapler. The two loops are, then, detubularized from the distal end to the operative holes, and the posterior baseplate of the VIP-n is reconfigured according to the Padua technique (Fig. 4.2) using a 3-0 barbed suture (Filbloc 90-day absorbable suture, Assut Europe, Rome, Italy).

In both reconfiguration techniques, the urethra is anastomosed to the neobladder by two 3-0 barbed sutures (Filbloc 90-day absorbable suture, Assut Europe, Rome, Italy), 20 cm for the right side and 15 cm for the left side, using the Van Velthoven technique (Fig. 4.3a, b) [54].

The 20-cm longer stitch is used to suture the right side of the urethra to the right hemi-circumference of the neobladder neck, and the first four stitches are used to reapproximate the urethra to the neobladder neck performing a posterior reconstruction by a modified "Rocco stitch" [55] sewing the posterior aspect of the

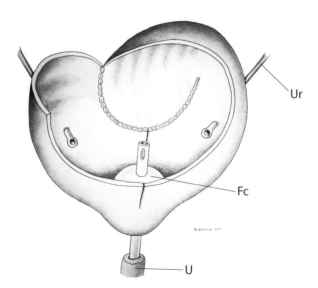

Fig. 4.2 A scheme of VIP-n reconstruction. The two distal third segments of the ileal loops are approximated, and, by a single charge of an Endo-GIA stapler, the distal funnel of the VIP-n is created. After detubularization of the ileum, the neobladder is tailored laparoscopically with a technique similar to "vescica ileale padovana" (*Ur* ureter, *Fc* Foley catheter, *U* urethra)

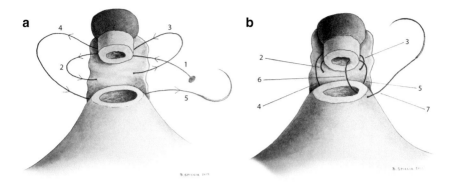

Fig. 4.3 (**a**) The figure shows the steps of the anastomosis between the neobladder funnel and the urethra, using two 3-0 barbed sutures (20 cm for the right side and 15 cm for the left side), by a Van Velthoven technique. The longer stitch is used to suture the right side of the urethra to the right hemi-circumference of the neobladder funnel. The first four stitches are used to reapproximate the urethra to the neobladder performing a posterior reconstruction by a modified "Rocco stitch" sewing the posterior aspect of the urethra to the residual Denonvilliers' fascia (1, 2, 3, 4, 5 = subsequent passages of the same suture). (**b**) The urethra and the neobladder funnel are progressively approximated (3, 4, 5, 6, 7 = subsequent passages of the same suture)

urethra to the residual Denonvilliers' fascia and the latter to the posterior aspect of the neobladder neck.

Each ureter is spatulated for a length of 2 cm and separately anastomosed to the terminal ends of the U-n ileal segment or laterally to the posterior baseplate of the VIP-n, using a simple Le Duc technique with continuous, 3-0 barbed sutures [56]. Two single-J, 7-Ch, 40-cm ureteral stents are inserted by a Seldinger technique using a 3-mm trocar or a MiniPort (Covidien) through the abdominal wall, at the midline, just above the symphysis [57]. Then the anterior aspect of the VIP-n or the operative opening of the U-n is closed with 3-0 Filbloc running sutures (Fig. 4.4).

The entire procedures are performed intracorporeally.

The reconstructed neobladder is irrigated at the end of the procedure to check a watertight closure, and any leak is secured with interrupted 2-0 Vicryl sutures. A drain is placed in the pelvis through a lateral port site.

The postoperative care includes removal of the nasogastric tube on postoperative day 1, pouch irrigation every 8 h starting on postoperative day 1, and removal of the abdominal drain when the output is <50 mL/day. The ureteral stents are removed 9 days postoperatively. The catheter is removed at 3 weeks if no leak is observed by a contrast medium evaluation.

In our experience [45] none of the treated cases was converted to open surgery, and we didn't have any perioperative mortalities. The median operating time was 365 min, with a median blood loss of 290 mL, a transfusion rate of 26.6%, and median hospital staying of 9 days. Patients with non-organ-confined disease or positive lymph nodes received adjuvant chemotherapy.

According to the modified Clavien classification system [58], 26.2% of patients had early complications, majority of them (87,5%) presenting low-grade complications (Clavien grades 1–2). Late complications occurred in 30% of patients

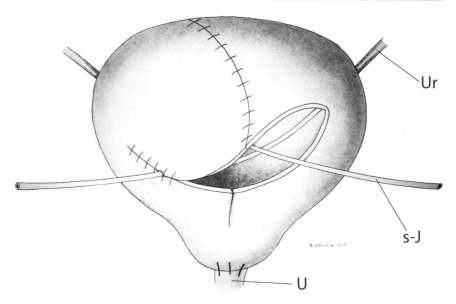

Fig. 4.4 A schematic scheme of VIP-reconstruction. After the ureteral-ileal and the urethral-neobladder anastomoses, the anterior aspect of the neobladder is closed with the two single-J, placed in the ureter passing through the neobladder wall (*Ur* ureter, *U* urethra, *s-J* ureteral stent)

(two pts Clavien grade 3b). Low-grade complications occurred more frequently during the first 20 days postoperatively and significantly earlier when compared to high-grade complications. All high-grade complications occurred after at least 32 days. The functional outcomes, specifically related to U-n reconstruction, were assessed by means of clinical and videourodynamic evaluation at 180 from surgery [59]. Daytime and nightime continence rates were 83.3 % and 73.3 %, respectively. The mean maximal neobladder capacity was 295 mL, with a mean post-void residual volume of 54 (range, 0–220) mL and a peak flow rate of 13.6 (9.7–33) mL/s. Three patients needed intermittent self-catheterization for significant chronic urinary retention (>150 mL). All these patients were also submitted to a rigorous oncologic follow-up (median 16.5 months, range 9–32). Eleven patients completed 2 years of follow-up. At the last outpatient visit, 73.3 % of pts were alive without evidence of recurrence, 6 % of pts had both local recurrence and distant metastases, 3 % of pts had only local recurrence, and 3 % of pts had only distant metastasis. 16.6 % of pts died from various causes (metastases, causes unrelated to the bladder cancer such as myocardial infarction or from a car accident).

The functional follow-up of the VIP-n cohort is still ongoing, and therefore long-term results are not still available.

4.3.3   Considerations

Mini-invasive surgery has considerably improved over the last decade, with indications now including difficult and prolonged procedures, such as RC [50, 60] with orthotopic neobladder reconstruction.

There is a significant variability in the results reported by various authors which reflects the difference in surgical expertise and the volume of performed procedures; this causes a lack of a consensus about the surgical technique and type of UD that can be preferable in laparoscopic surgery [61].

However data from literature support the laparoscopic management of localized MIBC and show acceptable operating time, intraoperative blood loss, hospitalization, and overall complication rate.

Furthermore, recently some experiences with RC and UD performed by robotic approach have been published with encouraging results. In a prospective, comparative analysis between LRC and RARC with ileal conduit, Abraham et al. reported that both LRC and RARC can be safely performed without compromising oncologic standards for surgical margins or the extent of LND. The robotic approach appeared to have a shorter learning curve and to be associated with less blood loss, fewer complications, and an earlier return of bowel function than LRC [62].

Long-term oncologic and functional results of LRC and RARC are still not comparable with those described in the case series of pts treated by open technique, being the experience with the mini-invasive approaches still limited in terms of population, length of follow-up, and surgical centers routinely performing these techniques.

All these data should prompt the use of the mini-invasive approaches to perform RC and UD. In fact, compared to the open procedure, these techniques have three principal advantages:

- *Better operative view*: this facilitates meticulous dissection and reduces injury to the pelvic floor structure improving the early postoperative recovery of continence.
- *Good hemostasis*: the pneumo-peritoneal pressure contributes to reduce blood leakage.
- *No extracorporeal bowel exposure*: this determines quicker postoperative functional recovery of the intestinal tract and decreases the incidence of related postoperative complications.

All the laparoscopic and robotic surgeons agree that LRC as RARC with totally intracorporeal UD are procedures for trained equips and that a significant laparoscopic experience is mandatory to reduce the operative time and complication rate. Furthermore, patient selection, surgical strategy, and use of specific devices can be crucial to simplify some of the critical steps of these procedures. These aspects are essential to shorten the operation, which is mostly dedicated to the reconstructive phase.

Of course, even if the experiences already reported in literature encourage the adoption of mini-invasive approaches to perform RC and UD, large cohort prospective randomized multicentric studies are still lacking to produce unequivocal scientific evidence.

References

1. Goossens-Laan CA, Visser O, Hulshof MC, et al. Survival after treatment for carcinoma invading bladder muscle: a Dutch population-based study on the impact of hospital volume. BJUInt. 2012;110:226–32.

2. Babjuk M, Burger M, Zigeuner R, Shariat SF, Van Rhijn BW, Compérat E, Sylvester RJ, Kaasinen E, Böhle A, Palou Redorta J, Rouprêt M. EAU guidelines on non-muscle-invasive urothelial carcinoma of the bladder: update 2013. European Association of Urology. Eur Urol. 2013;64(4):639–53. doi: 10.1016/j.eururo.2013.06.003. Epub 2013 Jun 12. Review.
3. Hautmann RE, Abol-Enein H, Hafez K, Haro I, Mansson W, Mills RD, Montie JD, Sagalowsky AI, Stein JP, Stenzl A, Studer UE, Volkmer BG. World Health Organization (WHO) consensus conference in bladder cancer, urinary diversion. Urology. 2007;69(1 Suppl):17–49.
4. Lebret T, Herve JM, Yonneau L, et al. After cystectomy, is it justified to perform a bladder replacement for patients with lymph node positive bladder cancer? Eur Urol. 2002; 42(4):344–9.
5. Stein JP, Lieskovsky G, Cote R, Groshen S, Feng AC, Boyd S, Skinner E, Bochner B, Thangathurai D, Mikhail M, Raghavan D, Skinner DG. Radical cystectomy in the treatment of invasive bladder cancer: long-term results in 1,054 patients. J Clin Oncol. 2001;19(3): 666–75.
6. Witjes JA, Compérat E, Cowan NC, De Santis M, Gakis G, Lebret T, Ribal MJ, Van der Heijden AG, Sherif A. European Association of Urology. Eur Urol. 2014;65(4):778–92. doi: 10.1016/j.eururo.2013.11.046. Epub 2013 Dec 12.
7. Miller DC, Taub DA, Dunn RL, et al. The impact of co-morbid disease on cancer control and survival following radical cystectomy. J Urol. 2003;169(1):105–9.
8. Extermann M, Overcash J, Lyman GH, et al. Comorbidity and functional status are independent in older cancer patients. J Clin Oncol. 1998;16(4):1582–7.
9. Ashworth A. Papillomatosis of the urethra. Br J Urol. 1956;28(1):3–13.
10. Raz S, Mclorie G, Johnson S, Skinner DG. Management of the urethra in patients undergoing radical cystectomy for bladder carcinoma. J Urol. 1978;120(3):298–300.
11. Faysal MH. Urethrectomy in men with transitional cell carcinoma of bladder. Urology. 1980;16(1):23–6.
12. Hardeman SW, Soloway MS. Urethral recurrence following radical cystectomy. J Urol. 1990;144(3):666–9.
13. Levinson AK, Johnson DE, Wishnow KI. Indications for urethrectomy in an era of continent urinary diversion. J Urol. 1990;144(1):73–5.
14. Tobisu K, Tanaka Y, Mizutani T, Kakizoe T. Transitional cell carcinoma of the urethra in men following cystectomy for bladder cancer: multivariate analysis for risk factors. J Urol. 1991;146(6):1551–3; discussion 1553-4.
15. Nieder AM, Sved PD, Gomez P, Kim SS, Manoharan M, Soloway MS. Urethral recurrence after cystoprostatectomy: implications for urinary diversion and monitoring. Urology. 2004; 64(5):950–4.
16. Stein JP, Clark P, Miranda G, Cai J, Groshen S, Skinner DG. Urethral tumor recurrence following cystectomy and urinary diversion: clinical and pathological characteristics in 768 male patients. J Urol. 2005;173(4):1163–8.
17. Stenzl A, Draxl H, Posch B, Colleselli K, Falk M, Bartsch G. The risk of urethral tumors in female bladder cancer: can the urethra be used for orthotopic reconstruction of the lower urinary tract? J Urol. 1995;153(3 Pt 2):950–5.
18. Freeman JA, Tarter TA, Esrig D, Stein JP, Elmajian DA, Chen SC, Groshen S, Lieskovsky G, Skinner DG. Urethral recurrence in patients with orthotopic ileal neobladders. J Urol. 1996;156(5):1615–9.
19. Hassan JM, Cookson MS, Smith Jr JA, Chang SS. Urethral recurrence in patients following orthotopic urinary diversion. J Urol. 2004;172(4 Pt 1):1338–41.
20. Wood Jr DP, Montie JE, Pontes JE, Levin HS. Identification of transitional cell carcinoma of the prostate in bladder cancer patients: a prospective study. J Urol. 1989;142(1):83–5.
21. Sakamoto N, Tsuneyoshi M, Naito S, Kumazawa J. An adequate sampling of the prostate to identify prostatic involvement by urothelial carcinoma in bladder cancer patients. J Urol. 1993;149(2):318–21.
22. Lebret T, Hervé JM, Barré P, Gaudez F, Lugagne PM, Barbagelatta M, Botto H. Urethral recurrence of transitional cell carcinoma of the bladder. Predictive value of preoperative lateromontanal biopsies and urethral frozen sections during prostatocystectomy. Eur Urol. 1998;33(2):170–4.

23. Donat SM, Wei DC, McGuire MS, Herr HW. The efficacy of transurethral biopsy for predicting the long-term clinical impact of prostatic invasive bladder cancer. J Urol. 2001;165(5):1580–4.
24. Azimuddin K, Khubchandani IT, Stasik JJ, et al. Neoplasia after ureterosigmoidostomy. Dis Colon Rectum. 1999;42(12):1632–8.
25. Stein JP, Cote RJ, Freeman JA, Esrig D, Elmajian DA, Groshen S, Skinner EC, Boyd SD, Lieskovsky G, Skinner DG. Indications for lower urinary tract reconstruction in women after cystectomy for bladder cancer: a pathological review of female cystectomy specimens. J Urol. 1995;154(4):1329–33.
26. Maralani S, Wood Jr DP, Grignon D, Banerjee M, Sakr W, Pontes JE. Incidence of urethral involvement in female bladder cancer: an anatomic pathologic study. Urology. 1997;50(4): 537–41.
27. Stein JP, Esrig D, Freeman JA, Grossfeld GD, Ginsberg DA, Cote RJ, Groshen S, Boyd SD, Lieskovsky G, Skinner DG. Prospective pathologic analysis of female cystectomy specimens: risk factors for orthotopic diversion in women. Urology. 1998;51(6):951–5.
28. Stein JP, Ginsberg DA, Skinner DG. Indications and technique of the orthotopic neobladder in women. Urol Clin North Am. 2002;29(3):725–34, xi.
29. Lance RS, Dinney CP, Swanson D, Babaian RJ, Pisters LL, Palmer LJ, Grossman HB. Radical cystectomy for invasive bladder cancer in the octogenarian. Oncol Rep. 2001;8(4):723–6.
30. Clark PE, Stein JP, Groshen SG, Cai J, Miranda G, Lieskovsky G, Skinner DG. Radical cystectomy in the elderly: comparison of clinical outcomes between younger and older patients. Cancer. 2005;104(1):36–43.
31. Sogni F, Brausi M, Frea B, Martinengo C, Faggiano F, Tizzani A, Gontero P. Morbidity and quality of life in elderly patients receiving ileal conduit or orthotopic neobladder after radical cystectomy for invasive bladder cancer. Urology. 2008;71(5):919–23. doi:10.1016/j.urology.2007.11.125. Epub 2008 Mar 20.
32. Elmajian DA, Stein JP, Skinner DG. Orthotopic urinary diversion: the Kock ileal neobladder. World J Urol. 1996;14(1):40–6.
33. Dutta SC, Chang SC, Coffey CS, Smith Jr JA, Jack G, Cookson MS. Health related quality of life assessment after radical cystectomy: comparison of ileal conduit with continent orthotopic neobladder. J Urol. 2002;168:164–7.
34. Porter MP, Penson DF. Health related quality of life after radical cystectomy and urinary diversion for bladder cancer: a systematic review and critical analysis of the literature. J Urol. 2005;173:1318–22.
35. Siracusano S, Niero M, Lonardi C, Cerruto MA, Ciciliato S, Toffoli L, Visalli F, Massidda D, Iafrate M, Artibani W, Bassi P, Imbimbo C, Racioppi M, Talamini R, D'Elia C, Cacciamani G, De Marchi D, Silvestri T, Verze P, Belgrano E. Development of a questionnaire specifically for patients with ileal orthotopic neobladder (IONB). Health Qual Life Outcomes. 2014;12:135.
36. Imbimbo C, Mirone V, Siracusano S, Niero M, Cerruto MA, Lonardi C, Artibani W, Bassi P, Iafrate M, Racioppi M, Talamini R, Ciciliato S, Toffoli L, Visalli F, Massidda D, D'Elia C, Cacciamani G, De Marchi D, Silvestri T, Creta M, Belgrano E, Verze P. Urology. 2015 Aug 17. Quality of life assessment with orthotopic ileal neobladder reconstruction after radical cystectomy: results from a prospective Italian multicenter observational study].
37. Hautmann RE. Urinary diversion: ileal conduit to neobladder. J Urol. 2003;169(3):834–42.
38. Abbas F, Biyabani SR, Talati J. Orthotopic bladder replacement to the urethra following salvage radical cystoprostatectomy in men with failed radiation therapy. Tech Urol. 2001;7(1): 20–6.
39. Ahlering TE, Kanellos A, Boyd SD, Lieskovsky G, Skinner DG, Bernstein L. A comparative study of perioperative complications with Kock pouch urinary diversion in highly irradiated versus nonirradiated patients. J Urol. 1988;139(6):1202–4.
40. Gschwend JE, May F, Paiss T, Gottfried HW, Hautmann RE. High-dose pelvic irradiation followed by ileal neobladder urinary diversion: complications and long-term results. Br J Urol. 1996;77(5):680–3.
41. Bochner BH, Figueroa AJ, Skinner EC, Lieskovsky G, Petrovich Z, Boyd SD, Skinner DG. Salvage radical cystoprostatectomy and orthotopic urinary diversion following radiation failure. J Urol. 1998;160(1):29–33.

42. Nieuwenhuijzen JA, Horenblas S, Meinhardt W, van Tinteren H, Moonen LM. Salvage cystectomy after failure of interstitial radiotherapy and external beam radiotherapy for bladder cancer. BJU Int. 2004;94(6):793–7.
43. Huang EY, Skinner EC, Boyd SD, Cai J, Miranda G, Daneshmand S. Radical cystectomy with orthotopic neobladder reconstruction following prior radical prostatectomy. World J Urol. 2012;30(6):741–5. doi:10.1007/s00345-012-0861-x. Epub 2012 Mar 29.
44. Urs E Studer, Richard E. Hautmann, M Hohenfellner, Robert D Mills, Yusaku Okada, Randall G. Rowland, Kenichi Tobisu, Taiji Tsukamoto. Indications for continent diversion after cystectomy and factors affecting long-term results Received: February 5, 1999.
45. Pastore AL, Palleschi G, Silvestri L, Cavallaro G, Rizzello M, Silecchia G, de Nunzio C, Al-Rawashdah SF, Petrozza V, Carbone A. Pure intracorporeal laparoscopic radical cystectomy with orthotopic "U" shaped ileal neobladder. BMC Urol. 2014;14:89. doi:10.1186/1471-2490-14-89.
46. Porpiglia F, Renard J, Billia M, Scoffone C, Cracco A, Terrone C, Scarpa RM. Open versus laparoscopy assisted radical cystectomy: results of a prospective study. J Endourol. 2007;21:325–9. doi:10.1089/end.2006.0224.
47. Huang J, Lin T, Xu K, Huang H, Jiang C, Han J, Yao Y, Guo Z, Xie W, Yin X, Zhang C. Laparoscopic radical cystectomy with orthotopic ileal neobladder: a report of 85 cases. J Endourol. 2008;22:939–46. doi:10.1089/end.2007.0298.
48. Parra RO, Andrus CH, Jones JP, Boullier JA. Laparoscopic cystectomy: initial report on a new treatment for the retained bladder. J Urol. 1992;148:1140–4.
49. Pastore AL, Palleschi G, Silvestri L, Leto A, Sacchi K, Pacini L, Petrozza V, Carbone A. Prospective randomized study of radiofrequency versus ultrasound scalpels on functional outcomes of laparoscopic radical prostatectomy. J Endourol. 2013;27:989–93. doi:10.1089/end.2013.0033.
50. Gill IS, Fergany A, Klein EA, Kaouk JH, Sung GT, Meraney AM, Savage SJ, Ulchaker JC, Novick AC. Laparoscopic radical cystoprostatectomy with ileal conduit performed completely intracorporeally: the initial 2 cases. Urology. 2000;56:26–9. doi:10.1016/S0090-4295(00)00598-7.
51. Wang GJ, Barocas DA, Raman JD, Scherr DS. Robotic vs open radical cystectomy: prospective comparison of perioperative outcomes and pathological measures of early oncological efficacy. BJU Int. 2008;101:89–93.
52. Pruthi RS, Wallen EM. Robotic assisted laparoscopic radical cystoprostatectomy: operative and pathological outcomes. J Urol. 2007;178:814–8. doi:10.1016/j.juro.2007.05.040.
53. Hasson HM, Rotman C, Rana N, Kumari NA. Open laparoscopy: 29-year experience. Obstet Gynecol. 2000;96:763–6. doi:10.1016/S0029-7844(00)01026-7.
54. Van Velthoven RF, Ahlering TE, Peltier A, Skarecky DW, Clayman RV. Technique for laparoscopic running urethrovesical anastomosis: the single knot method. Urology. 2003;61:699–702. doi:10.1016/S0090-4295(02)02543-8.
55. Spinelli MG, Cozzi G, Grasso A, Talso M, Varisco D, Abed El Rahman D, Acquati P, Albo G, Rocco B, Maggioni A, Rocco F. Ralp and Rocco stitch: original technique. Urologia. 2011;18(78 Suppl):35–8. doi:10.5301/RU.2011.8773.
56. Bricker EM. Bladder substitution after pelvic evisceration. Surg Clin North Am. 1950;30:1511–21.
57. Seldinger SI. Catheter replacement of the needle in percutaneous arteriography; a new technique. Acta Radiol. 1953;39:368–76. doi:10.3109/00016925309136722.
58. Dindo D, Demartines N, Clavien PA. Classification of surgical complications: a new proposal with evaluation in a cohort of 6336 patients and results of a survey. Ann Surg. 2004;240(2):205–13.
59. Palleschi G, Pastore AL, Ripoli A, Silvestri L, Petrozza V, Carbone A. Videourodynamic evaluation of intracorporeally reconstructed orthotopic U-shaped ileal neobladders. Urology. 2015;85(4):883–9.
60. Puppo P, Naselli A. Laparoscopic radical cystectomy. Where do we stand? Arch Esp Urol. 2010;63:508–19. doi:10.4321/S0004-06142010000700005.

61. Aboumarzouk OM, Drewa T, Olejniczak P, Chlosta PL. Laparoscopic versus open radical cystectomy for muscle-invasive bladder cancer: a single institute comparative analysis. Urol Int. 2013;91(1):109–12. doi:10.1159/000350237.
62. Abraham JB, Young JL, Box GN, Lee HJ, Deane LA, Ornstein DK. Comparative analysis of laparoscopic and robot-assisted radical cystectomy with ileal conduit urinary diversion. J Endourol. 2007;21(12):1473–80. doi:10.1089/end.2007.0095.

Robot-Assisted Radical Cystectomy and Totally Intracorporeal Urinary Diversions

5

Giuseppe Simone, Michele Gallucci, and Inderbir Gill

5.1 Background

Minimally invasive approaches have dramatically modified perioperative outcomes of most urological surgical procedures. The development and standardization of laparoscopic radical prostatectomy have significantly reduced perioperative blood loss and transfusion rates. A review by Novara et al. demonstrated that robot-assisted radical prostatectomy further reduced perioperative transfusion rates compared with the laparoscopic approach [1].

Similarly, laparoscopic radical nephrectomy has been acknowledged as the standard of care for most cT2-3 kidney neoplasms thanks to its significant impact on perioperative outcomes [2].

Available evidences from one randomized clinical trial (RCT) [3] and from two nonrandomized studies [4, 5] showed a significantly shorter hospital stay and lower analgesic requirement for the laparoscopic radical nephrectomy (RN) group compared with the open group. One of these studies also reported shorter convalescence [5]. All these studies reported significantly lower perioperative blood in the laparoscopic arms [3–5].

In the only prospective randomized study comparing laparoscopic versus open nephroureterectomy for upper urinary tract urothelial carcinoma, laparoscopic approach was significantly associated with reduced blood loss and shorter hospitalization (both p values <0.001) [6].

G. Simone (✉) • M. Gallucci
Department of Urology, "Regina Elena" National Cancer Institute, Rome, Italy
e-mail: puldet@gmail.com

I. Gill
Catherine and Joseph Aresty Department of Urology, USC Institute of Urology,
Keck School of Medicine, University of Southern California, Los Angeles, CA, USA

© Springer International Publishing Switzerland 2016
A. Carbone et al. (eds.), *Functional Urologic Surgery in Neurogenic and Oncologic Diseases*, Urodynamics, Neurourology and Pelvic Floor Dysfunctions, DOI 10.1007/978-3-319-29191-8_5

On the contrary, with regard to radical cystectomy, perioperative morbidity, high-grade complication, and mortality rates of contemporary open radical cystectomy (ORC) series remain remarkable, with the overall complication rate ranging between 19 and 64 % in different series [7]. In a contemporary prospective multi-institutional series, the incidence of severe (grade ≥3 Clavien) complications approached 14 % [8]. Most of these complications were not due to cystectomy itself while depending on the need to perform a meticulous pelvic lymph node dissection and, moreover, to create a urinary diversion (UD) using ileal or colonic segments. These steps require advanced surgical skills for intracorporeal sutures and remain time-consuming also for highly experienced surgeons. To reduce the morbidity of this procedure, as well as to latch on to the growing wave of minimally invasive surgery that has swept through urology in the past two decades, robotic-assisted radical cystectomy has gained interests in the past several years [9].

Radical cystectomy (RC) consists of three main steps: cystectomy, pelvic lymph node dissection (PLND), and finally urinary diversion (UD). The complexity of this procedure and, consequently, the perioperative complications are mainly related to the last surgical step. Notably, each one of these three steps is a complex surgical step itself; thus, performing the first two is certainly time-consuming and technically demanding, especially at the beginning of the learning curve. As a result, in the development era of minimally invasive RC, UD was performed extracorporeally, in order to minimize the need for intracorporeal sutures, and besides it is reasonable to think that there was an overuse of incontinent urinary diversion due to the advanced skills required to perform either orthotopic or continent cutaneous UDs.

This process has not been free of consequences, since the goal of mini-invasive radical cystectomy (MIRC) should be undoubtedly a totally intracorporeal surgical procedure that has provided the known benefits reported above for other urologic procedures in terms of reduced intraoperative blood loss, accelerated recovery of patients, and minimal cosmetic impact. Whether this would turn into a significant clinical benefit for patients has not yet been established and is beyond the scope of this text.

The aim of this chapter is the description of surgical steps of different UDs performed with robot assistance and an overview of available reports on perioperative and functional outcomes of published series.

5.2   Surgical Technique

Robot-assisted radical cystectomy (RARC) is a major urologic surgery. The first steps of this procedure consist on the removal of the bladder along with prostate and seminal vesicles in men and with uterus and ovaries in female patients. Usually, the PLND is performed as second step. A steep Trendelenburg position is specifically required for these first two steps only, in order to guarantee an adequate view of the surgical field. Later in the last step, the position is changed to 15° Trendelenburg, since a steep

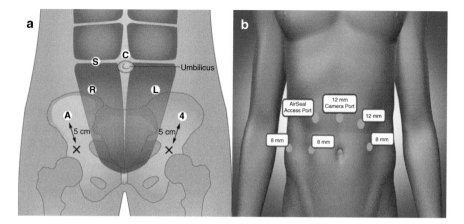

Fig. 5.1 (**a**, **b**) Alternative options for ports' placement

position is not necessary for the accomplishment of UDs and may seldom contrast a tension-free anastomosis between the neobladder and the urethral stump.

5.2.1   Port Placement

In a review by Azzouni, the port placement was summarized as follows (Fig. 5.1a): at point C, a periumbilical 12 mm port is placed for the camera. Three 8 mm ports are placed at the right and left edges of the rectus abdominis (R and L) below the level of the umbilicus and approximately 5 cm above the left anterior superior iliac spine (position 4) for the right, left, and fourth robotic arms, respectively. At position A, a 15 mm port is placed approximately 5 cm cranial to the right anterior superior iliac spine for passage of the Endo GIA™ stapler by the bedside assistant. A 5 mm port is placed midway between the camera and right robotic arm ports (position S) to be used by the bedside assistant for the passage of the laparoscopic suction/irrigation device. Basically, following this approach, the assistant works on the left bedside with a 5 mm port for the left hand and a 15 mm port for the right hand [10].

The following picture (Fig. 5.1b), instead, highlights an alternative port placement as reported by Papalia et al. [11].

The 12 mm camera port is placed more cranially, midway between the umbilicus and the xiphoid process. Essentially, the position of the camera port depends on the surgeon preference about the extent of PLND. The higher is the camera port the easier will be the exposure of aortic bifurcation during the PLND.

This port placement allows the assistant to work with two 12 mm ports, one for each side. This is essentially done to allow him to have an easier access and a more comfortable use of motorized robotic staplers either for the management of both bladder pedicles or for the ileal resection and its side to side anastomosis or for the stapling of the orthotopic neobladder. An additional suprapubic MiniPort was placed to introduce guidewires and double-J stents.

5.2.2 Cystectomy

The goal of this surgical step is to remove the bladder entirely, avoiding any viola-tion of urinary tract and achieving negative soft tissue surgical margins.

The prevention of any urine leakage during the procedure is mandatory in order to minimize the risk of tumor seeding into either the pelvic or the peritoneal cavity. Therefore, the respect of bladder integrity and a careful dissection of the urethral stump are key steps of an oncologically sound procedure. For this reason the ure-thral catheter is pulled back, and a Weck clip is applied in order to maintain the catheter balloon in tight junction with the bladder neck.

The growing interest in performing "organ sparing" and "sex sparing" proce-dures has led to the development of conservative options either in male or in female patients undergoing RC. Since the description of these techniques would be beyond the scope of this text, we will quickly summarize these options and report some preliminary unpublished intraoperative pictures to support the feasi-bility of them.

In male patients nerve-sparing RC has demonstrated to provide satisfactory func-tional outcomes with comparable oncologic efficacy in open series. Multiple options to spare the prostate gland, either partially or entirely, have been reported. All these techniques have certainly a positive impact on the sexual function preservation, although some authors have reported inferior oncologic outcomes in terms of local recurrence and distant metastasis rate [12, 13].

Sex-sparing RC in female patients is a viable option in young patients, especially for anteriorly located tumors where the total preservation of vagina does not affect cancer control. Several reports have supported feasibility, perioperative safety, and optimal functional outcomes in selected patient populations.

5.2.3 Pelvic Lymph Node Dissection

This surgical step is an integral part of the procedures. Omitting this procedure undermines staging accuracy and cancer control [14].

Despite a wide literature supporting the need for a meticulous PLND [15], pos-sibly extended up to the aortic bifurcation [16], the optimal extent of PLND is still under investigation. Two ongoing prospective randomized trials will hopefully pro-vide strong evidence in this field [17, 18].

The important message for readers is that robotic approach has demonstrated, since the development era, to provide adequate lymph node yield compared to open series. A meticulous PLND is feasible and safe during RARC and does not affect the entire duration of surgical procedure (60–75 min for an extended and a superex-tended template, respectively).

An intraoperative view of the surgical field following an extended PLND is depicted in Fig. 5.2. It is clearly visible the aortic bifurcation, the presacral space completely dissected out from fat/lymphatic tissue and the iliac bifurcations.

Fig. 5.2 Intraoperative view of extended pelvic lymph node dissection template (upper boundary at aortic bifurcation, complete dissection of presacral nodes)

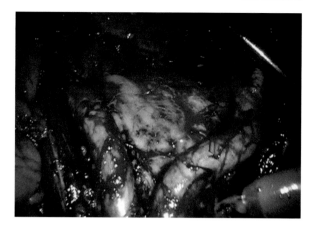

5.2.4 Urinary Diversion

The best candidates for ileal conduit, for orthotopic neobladder, or for continent cutaneous diversion are yet to be established. The WHO consensus has clearly highlighted that "the primary patient factor is the patient's desire for a neobladder." Obviously, there are some absolute contraindications to orthotopic neobladder, including compromised renal function, disease location and extent requiring simultaneous urethrectomy, and severe hepatic and intestinal function (i.e., inflammatory bowel disease). Keeping in mind the absolute ones, the relative contraindications include poor performance status and urethral strictures, which should be carefully considered during patients counseling.

Continent cutaneous diversions (CCDs) are complex surgical procedures; the use of such options has some contraindications, such as the lack of manual dexterity, which could affect the ability of patients to perform self-catheterization. These options are commonly reserved to young female patients unfit for neobladder while highly motivated to avoid an incontinent stoma.

However, a real benefit of either orthotopic neobladder or CCDs over the ileal conduit in terms of patients' quality of life (QoL) has not been demonstrated, and ileal conduit certainly represents the most commonly used UD [19].

Published evidence does not support an advantage of one type of reconstruction over the others with regard to QoL. An important reason is probably that patients are subjected preoperatively to method-to-patient matching and thus are prepared for disadvantages and advantages associated with different methods.

5.2.4.1 Orthotopic Neobladder

Regardless of multiple orthotopic reservoirs described, in this text we will report about the totally intracorporeal Studer and Padua ileal neobladder models. Both these neobladders are created according to the milestone principles of detubularization and cross-folding of the ileum to guarantee a globular shape and a low-pressure reservoir.

Studer Pouch [20]

The surgical steps of the open Studer pouch were integrally replicated with a total intracorporeal approach by the University of Southern California team. Approximately 60 cm of the distal ileum (44 cm for the pouch, 16 cm for the chimney) is chosen, about 15 cm proximal to the ileocecal junction.

Two symmetrically aligned 22 cm ileal segments adjacent to each other are provisionally fixed to the urethral stump and the additional 15 cm of the ileum are used for the afferent limb as originally described by Studer et al. The 44 cm of the ileum, comprising the neobladder, is detubularized and the opposing edges of the posterior neobladder wall are aligned with several stay sutures and sutured in a watertight manner with 2-0 running barbed sutures. Once the posterior plate is complete, it is rotated 90° counterclockwise with caudal traction applied to the 3-0 suture to set up the urethroileal anastomosis. The distal Denonvilliers' fascia is then approximated to the rectourethralis muscle to reduce tension on the urethroileal anastomosis.

The urethroileal anastomosis is performed in a running fashion with a double-armed 3-0 Monocryl suture starting at the 6 o'clock position. With the posterior plate anastomosed to the urethra, secondary folding is accomplished by placing a midpoint horizontal mattress suture that divides the anterior suture line into two equal halves and aligns the edges for suturing. The anterior wall of the neobladder is closed with running 2-0 barbed sutures. A small opening is left in the anterior suture line to allow passage of bilateral ileoureteral stents and accomplishment of ureteroileal anastomoses. Each ureter is spatulated and separately anastomosed to the afferent limb using the Bricker technique with continuous 4-0 Vicryl sutures.

After suturing the posterior wall, a 7F, single-J, ileoureteral stent is inserted through a suprapubic 2 mm MiniPort trocar, internalized, and secured to the urethral catheter with nonabsorbable sutures to facilitate stent removal approximately 3 weeks postoperatively.

Finally, the anterior closure of the pouch is completed in a running fashion using barbed sutures.

Padua Ileal Bladder

The most declive part of the ileum is chosen, at a variable distance (minimum 20 cm) from the ileocecal valve with a length of about 42 cm. The division of the proximal ileum is made utilizing a single 60 mm stapler load, while the isolation of the distal extremity of the ileal segment is carried out with a 6–8 cm deep section of the "mesentery" using two consecutive stapler loads (60–45 mm).

The optimal point of the selected bowel loop to create the neobladder neck is identified about 12–14 cm proximally to the distal ileal section edge after ensuring a tension-free approach to the urethral stump.

The proximal half of the loop will configure the left base and the dome of the neobladder.

Ileal segments utilized to tailor the neobladder are the following:

- 10 cm for the neck configuration

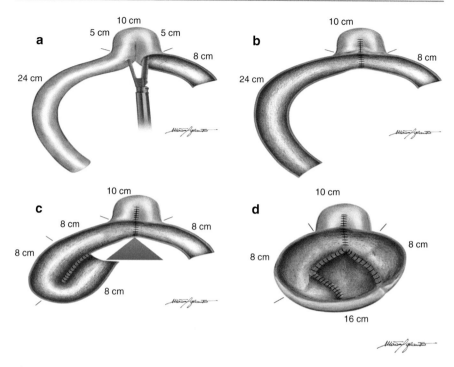

Fig. 5.3 (**a–d**) Main surgical steps of intracorporeal "vescica ileale padovana"

A triangle having 8 cm length sides with the vertex at the neobladder neck:

- 8 cm for the right plate
- 8 cm for the left plate
- A "U" folded 16 cm, resulting in an 8 cm segment for the dome

A 10 cm inverted U-shaped neobladder neck is created with a stay suture approximating the ileum segment at 8 and 18 cm far from the distal ileum border.

After detubularizing the 8 cm of the distal ileum along the antimesenteric border, motorized stapler arms are introduced through the two branches of the inverted U-shaped neobladder neck to approximate them and create the neobladder neck (Fig. 5.3a).

Two stapler loads are required to detubularize and suture simultaneously the 10 cm (5 + 5) of the ileum that structured the neck of the neobladder.

Subsequently, the remaining 24 cm of the ileum are detubularized starting from the proximal ileal edge (Fig. 5.3b).

The neobladder was now shaped as an 8 cm side equilateral triangle with the vertex at the inverted U-shaped neobladder neck (Fig. 5.3c).

The right side of the triangle is formed by the distal detubularized 8 cm of the ileum.

The 8 cm proximally to the U-shaped neobladder neck, left unfolded, shape the left side of the triangle.

The base of the triangle is finally shaped with staplers, folding the proximal 16 cm of the ileal segment on itself and approximating the extremity of the folded segment to the right side of the triangle, thus creating the neobladder dome.

Once the reservoir is externally shaped, the inner borders of the triangle sides are hand-sewn and the neobladder completed (Fig. 5.3d).

The anastomosis between the neobladder neck and the urethral stump is performed according to a previously described technique, after cutting the reservoir in the most declive part of the neobladder neck [9]. A 22 ch hematuria catheter is used and the balloon is inflated with 5 cc of saline solution.

Ureters are spatulated and passed through the posterior aspect of the neobladder. Ureteroileal anastomoses are performed according to Le Duc/Camey technique with 4-0 Monocryl interrupted sutures. Guidewires and 7F double-J stents are introduced through a suprapubic 2 mm MiniPort.

Finally, the anterior aspect of the neobladder is hand-sewn with two serous-serous running sutures.

Ileal Conduit

Totally intracorporeal ileal conduit after RARC is certainly feasible, easier than orthotopic neobladder and widely reproducible with shorter learning curve. In a recent consensus panel held in Pasadena, a group of experts recommended to perform ileal conduit reconstructions only in the first 20–30 patients of the learning curve. This is essentially due to the high morbidity and to the significant risk of high-grade complications related to orthotopic UD. In a preliminary analysis of the first 100 patients treated with RARC and totally intracorporeal UD at "Regina Elena" National Cancer Institute, the incidence of high-grade complications (Clavien 3–5) in patients who received orthotopic neobladder was tenfold higher compared to those who received ileal conduit (unpublished data). Surgical steps of totally intracorporeal ileal conduit are exactly the same described in Chap. 4 about the laparoscopic approach.

Indiana Pouch

The so-called Indiana pouch (IP) is the most known and the only totally intracorporeal CCD reported in literature. Continent cutaneous diversions are established options after RC; however, due to the complexity of surgical procedure and to the relatively poor number of patient candidates to such diversion, to date there is only a single report by Goh et al. about a totally intracorporeal ileocolonic pouch.

We hereby describe surgical steps and preliminary perioperative outcomes of ten consecutive patients treated with totally intracorporeal RARC and IP (University of Southern California and "Regina Elena" National Cancer Institute).

RARC and PLND are performed with a six-trocar access. Two additional ports are placed and the robot is re-docked laterally with the patient in left flank position. The following steps are replicated from standard open surgical techniques:

- 10 cm of the distal ileum and 30 cm of the right colon are isolated.
- Ileocolonic anastomosis is performed with a motorized stapler through the 12 mm trocar on the right anterior axillary line.
- 30 cm of the right colon is isolated, incised along the medial tenia up to 3 cm from the ileocecal valve and "U" folded.
- The medial aspect of the folded colon is robotically sewn, and refluxing uretero-colonic anastomoses are performed on the posterior aspect of the pouch.
- Double-J ureteral stents are inserted through a 2 mm Miniport and secured to a 22-Fr hematuria catheter inserted through the appendix.
- After closing the anterior aspect of the pouch, a 16-Fr Foley catheter is inserted through the umbilicus and into the efferent ileal limb. The catheter balloon is then inflated with 10 cc and placed into the colonic pouch.
- The ileocecal valve is then reinforced with sutures, and a motorized stapler is inserted through the umbilicus to taper the efferent limb.
- Finally, the efferent limb is extracted and the stoma created at the umbilical site.

Median operative time was 60 min for cystectomy, 65 min for PLND, and 210 min for pouch construction. No transfusions of any kind were needed and there were no major complications (Clavien III–V). Median hospital stay was 9 days. Larger cohorts and longer follow-up are needed to confirm the feasibility of this technique in other centers and to assess oncologic and functional outcomes.

Ureteroileal Anastomoses
The lack of strong evidence to support a specific ureteroileal anastomosis over the others has led to the adoption of different techniques. A WHO consensus conference on UD has clearly highlighted the effectiveness and the positive benefits/complications ratio of simple end-to-side, freely refluxing ureterointestinal anastomosis to an afferent limb of a low-pressure orthotopic reconstruction compared to "conventional" antireflux procedures that are affected by higher complication and reoperation rates without providing any functional advantage [19].

5.3   Perioperative Outcomes

There is an increasing number of reports, unequivocally suggesting favorable perioperative outcomes of RARC. In a recent review, the mean/median estimated blood loss ranged between 200 and 430 mL [21].

In a two-institutional report on 132 orthotopic neobladders (the UD with the higher incidence of perioperative complications), Clavien grade I, II, III, IV, and V complications within 30 days were 7%, 25%, 13%, 2%, and 0%, respectively, and between 30 and 90 days were 5%, 9%, 11%, 1%, and 2%, respectively [22].

5.4   Oncologic Outcomes

The major concern about RARC is about its oncologic non-inferiority compared to the standard treatment that is open RC. There are evidences supporting the midterm oncologic effectiveness of RARC: recently, in a multicenter analysis of more than 700 patients treated in 11 institutions with RARC, Raza et al. reported 5-year recurrence-free survival (RFS), cancer-specific survival (CSS), and overall survival rates (OS) of 67 %, 75 %, and 50 %, respectively [23]. However, the relatively poor number of patients treated, with selection biases of a retrospective analysis and the lack of prospective randomized trials versus open RC, suggests caution when considering RARC equally effective as open RC in terms of oncologic outcomes. Another interesting report from Gandaglia et al. on 155 consecutive patients treated at a single center reported poorer RFS rate (53.7 %), with comparable CSS rate 73.5 % and higher OS rate (65.2 %) [24]. Although these differences may be partially due to small sample sizes, they highlight the important role of selection criteria for RARC in determining a 15.2 % difference in the OS rate, and, more interestingly, among those 46.4 % of patients who experienced disease recurrence, 4 % had peritoneal recurrence that is one of the warnings raised by detractors of RARC.

5.5   Follow-Up Strategies

Follow-up schedule after RC includes periodic visits, biochemical tests, and advanced imaging, such as CT and MRI. However, if such intensive follow-up schedule significantly impacts on patients, survival is still a matter of debate. Recently, Strope et al. nicely demonstrated that the receipt of follow-up care in the later follow-up period was associated with improved survival [HR 0.23, 95 % CI 0.15–0.35; 0.27, 95 % CI, 0.18–0.40; 0.47, 95 % CI, 0.31–0.71, low, middle, and high tertile of expenditures, respectively], while an intensive imaging follow-up, usually applied in the first 2–5 years after cystectomy, does not improve patients' survival. Instrumental variable analysis suggested only doctor visits and urine testing [HRs, 0.96 (0.93–0.99) and 0.95 (0.91–0.99), respectively] improved survival [25].

References

1. Novara G, Ficarra V, Rosen RC, et al. Systematic review and meta-analysis of perioperative outcomes and complications after robot-assisted radical prostatectomy. Eur Urol. 2012;62:431–52.
2. Ljungberg B, Bensalah K, Bex A, et al. Guidelines on renal cell carcinoma 2015. Eur Urol 2010;58:398-406. http://uroweb.org/wp-content/uploads/EAU-Guidelines-Renal-Cell-Cancer-2015-v2.pdf.
3. Peng B, Zheng J-H, Xu D-F, Ren J-Z. Retroperitoneal laparoscopic nephrectomy and open nephrectomy for radical treatment of renal cell carcinoma: a comparison of clinical outcomes. Acad J Second Mil Univ. 2006;27:1167–9.

4. Gratzke C, Seitz M, Bayrle F, et al. Quality of life and perioperative outcomes after retroperitoneoscopic radical nephrectomy (RN), open RN and nephron-sparing surgery in patients with renal cell carcinoma. BJU Int. 2009;104:470–5.

5. Hemal AK, Kumar A, Kumar R, et al. Laparoscopic versus open radical nephrectomy for large renal tumors: a long-term prospective comparison. J Urol. 2007;177:862–6.

6. Simone G, Papalia R, Guaglianone S, et al. Laparoscopic versus open nephroureterectomy: perioperative and oncologic outcomes from a randomised prospective study. Eur Urol. 2009; 56:520–6.

7. Liedberg F. Early complications and morbidity of radical cystectomy. Eur Urol Suppl. 2010;9:25–30.

8. De Nunzio C, Cindolo L, Leonardo C, et al. Analysis of radical cystectomy and urinary diversion complications with the Clavien classification system in an Italian real life cohort. EJSO. 2013;39:792–8.

9. Steinberg PL, Ghavamian R. Robotic-assisted radical cystectomy. Current technique and outcomes. Expert Rev Anticancer Ther. 2012;12:913–7.

10. Azzouni F. Current status of robot-assisted radical cystectomy for bladder cancer. Nat Rev Urol. 2012;9:573–82. doi:10.1038/nrurol.2012.144.

11. Papalia R, Simone G, Ferriero M, Mastroianni R, Guaglianone S, Gallucci M. V30 totally intracorporeal robot-assisted vescica ileale Padovana (VIP) using staplers: a stepwise approach. Eur Urol Suppl. 2015;193:e978.

12. Simone G, Papalia R, Leonardo C, et al. Prostatic capsule and seminal vesicle-sparing cystectomy: improved functional results, inferior oncologic outcome. Urology. 2008;72:162–6.

13. Hautmann RE, Stein JP. Neobladder with prostatic capsule and seminal-sparing cystectomy for bladder cancer: a step in a wrong direction. Urol Clin N Am. 2005;32:177–85.

14. Abdollah F, Sun M, Schmitges J, et al. Stage-specific impact of pelvic lymph node dissection on survival in patients with non-metastatic bladder cancer treated with radical cystectomy. BJU Int. 2012;109:1147–54.

15. Dorin RP, Daneshmand S, Eisenberg MS, et al. Lymph node dissection technique is more important than lymph node count in identifying nodal metastases in radical cystectomy patients: a comparative mapping study. Eur Urol. 2011;60:946–52.

16. Simone G, Papalia R, Ferriero M, et al. Stage-specific impact of extended versus standard pelvic lymph node dissection in radical cystectomy. Int J Urol. 2013;20:390–7.

17. swog.org (homepage on the Internet). SWOG S1011 bladder cancer trial: patient information. http://swog.org/patients/s1011/.

18. Association of Urogenital Oncology (AUO). Eingeschränkte vs Ausgedehnte lymphadenektomie LEA (Limited vs Extended lymphadenectomy LEA). In: ClinicalTrials.gov (website on the Internet). Bethesda: US National Library of Medicine. 2011. Updated 7 Sept 2011. (http://clinicaltrials.gov/ct2/show/NCT01215071).

19. Hautmann RE, Abol-Enein H, Hafe K, et al. Urinary diversion. Urology. 2007;69:17–49.

20. Goh AC, Gill IS, Lee DJ, et al. Robotic intracorporeal orthotopic ileal neobladder: replicating open surgical principles. Eur Urol. 2012;62:891–901.

21. Chan KG, Guru K, Wiklund P, et al. Pasadena robot-assisted radical cystectomy and urinary diversion: technical recommendations from the Pasadena consensus panel. Eur Urol. 2015;67:423–31.

22. Desai MM, Gill IS, de Castro Abreu AL, et al. Robotic intracorporeal orthotopic neobladder during radical cystectomy in 132 patients. J Urol. 2014;192:1734–40.

23. Raza SJ, Wilson T, Peabody JO, et al. Long-term oncologic outcomes following robot-assisted radical cystectomy: results from the international robotic cystectomy consortium. Eur Urol. 2015;68:721–8.

24. Gandaglia G, De Groote R, Geurts N, et al. Oncologic outcomes of robot-assisted radical cystectomy: results of a high-volume robotic center. J Endourol. 2015. In press.

25. Strope SA, Chang SH, Chen L, Sandhu G, Piccirillo JF, Schootman M. Survival impact of follow-up care after radical cystectomy for bladder cancer. J Urol. 2013;190:1698–703.

Treating Incontinence after Prostatectomy and Cystectomy: Role of Advanced Minimally Invasive Surgery

David T. Greenwald, Ryan W. Dobbs, Cristian Gozzi, and Simone Crivellaro

6.1 Brief Overview of Stress Urinary Incontinence Following Surgical Intervention

While male urinary incontinence may result from a variety of conditions including traumatic injuries, traumatic and acquired myelopathies, and congenital disorders affecting the nervous system, in the United States, the most common cause of incompetence of the external sphincter is due to complications following radical prostatectomy and cystoprostatectomy. The importance of the management of post-prostatectomy patients cannot be understated. Due to both the prevalence and favorable prognosis of organ-confined prostate cancer, these patients represent the single largest type of male cancer survivors, comprising over 40 % of all male cancer survivors in the United States and a group of greater than 2.7 million men [1]. Contemporary studies of treatment utilization have shown that for men with clinically organ-confined prostate cancer, approximately half will choose prostatectomy as their primary treatment [2]. Comparisons for the exact rates of postoperative urinary incontinence between studies are difficult due to different study populations, designs, and definitions for urinary incontinence. In part due to this variability, studies have reported an extremely broad range for the rate of post-prostatectomy incontinence from 2.5 to 87 % [3]; however, more contemporary advances in

D.T. Greenwald • R.W. Dobbs
Urology Resident, PGY 2nd, University of Illinois at Chicago, Chicago, IL, USA

C. Gozzi
Urology Department, University of Pisa – Italy, Pisa, Italy

S. Crivellaro (✉)
Urology Department, University of Illinois at Chicago, Chicago, IL, USA
e-mail: crivellaro76@hotmail.com

© Springer International Publishing Switzerland 2016
A. Carbone et al. (eds.), *Functional Urologic Surgery in Neurogenic and Oncologic Diseases*, Urodynamics, Neurourology and Pelvic Floor Dysfunctions, DOI 10.1007/978-3-319-29191-8_6

surgical techniques including the introduction of robot-assisted radical prostatectomy (RARP) as compared to the classical retropubic prostatectomy (RRP) have led to a number of studies [4–6] to report more favorable incontinence rates with minimally invasive surgery with published rates of incontinence at 1 year ranging from 4 to 31 % following RARP with a mean incontinence rate of 16 % utilizing a "no pad" definition for continence [6]. Some studies have suggested that this improvement may have important clinical implications to patients in regard to surgical treatment for urinary incontinence following RP. Carlsson et al. [7] performed a prospective analysis of 1,253 RARP and 485 RRP patients which demonstrated significantly lower rates of surgical intervention following prostatectomy with 0.5 % ($n=7$) of RARP patients requiring placement of an AUS, while 2.2 % ($n=11$) patients in the RRP cohort required surgical treatment.

A number of factors influence postoperative urinary incontinence following RP including surgical approach, specific surgical techniques, and patient factors [8]. In general, patients should be counseled to utilize pelvic floor muscle exercises following prostatectomy as well as to expect a progressive improvement in postoperative urinary continence following surgery [9–11]. Several randomized studies [12, 13] have demonstrated the effectiveness of pelvic floor rehabilitation following catheter removal as the first-line noninvasive treatment for post-prostatectomy incontinence. Electrical stimulation and biofeedback in conjunction with pelvic floor rehabilitation have been also evaluated; however, the results of these studies have not demonstrated an improvement in outcomes [14], and presently these adjuncts are not recommended in available guidelines [15]. While the majority of patients do regain continence, a subset of patients will have persistent urinary issues following surgery, and patients should be counseled that these symptoms may present several years following their initial treatment. At a 5-year follow-up, Penson et al. [16] noted 14 % of 1,288 men post-RRP reported frequent urinary leakage or no urinary control, a greater proportion than the 10 % of patients reporting similar symptoms at the 2-year follow-up. Similarly, a 10-year follow-up after RRP has shown declines in urinary function from 2 to 8 years and small but significant declines from 8 to 10 years [17]. While these declines may represent the consequences of aging in an elderly male population, they represent a significant clinical concern for both urologists and patients.

In the case of cystectomy and orthotopic neobladder, postoperative urinary incontinence can be attributed to many variables, including age, surgical indication, prior treatments (such as radiation or previous transurethral resection of the prostate), and specific surgical technique. There are many reported series which outline post-cystectomy incontinence, although they vary with their definition of incontinence, the technique used to collect information (chart review, telephone interview, anonymous questionnaire), and the length of follow-up [18].

Nearly all these series include a gradual improvement in daytime continence over the first 6–12 months post-op, and a persistent nighttime incontinence reported in 20–50 % of patients. Steers [19] reported an average daytime incontinence of 13 % from a pooled analysis for 2,238 patients with varying forms of orthotopic neobladder, with age over 65, the use of colonic segment, and lack of nerve-sparing technique as risk factors for incontinence. Results from a multivariate analysis of 331 male patients who underwent cystoprostatectomy with ileal neobladder corroborated that patients younger than 65 and those with nerve-sparing technique have a much higher rate of daytime continence [20]. Nerve-sparing technique, however, is less advantageous with bulkier tumors or tumors on the posterior bladder wall, trigone, or bladder neck due to increased risk of positive surgical margins (which can be fatal).

Nighttime incontinence is noted in an average 28 % of neobladders [19] – ranging 7–70 % – but generally improves over time as the functional capacity increases and the absorptive capacity of the mucosa improves – which is attributed to a reversal in the normal antidiuretic effect of nighttime [21]. Nighttime incontinence may improve as late as 24 months postoperatively [22, 23].

Orthotopic neobladder enlargement may take 6–12 months postcystoprostatectomy, until which the management of urinary incontinence should be delayed [23, 24]. Initial therapy of post-cystectomy incontinence includes physical therapy with biofeedback focused on pelvic floor muscles [25]. Urodynamics may be utilized to assess neobladder capacity and evaluate for a reduction in maximal urethral closure (or low Valsalva leak pressure) – in which situation transurethral bulking agents may be considered for mild incontinence. Artificial urethral sphincter provides more definitive management of moderate to severe post-cystoprostatectomy incontinence [26].

For patients with persistent or severe urinary incontinence who demonstrate no improvement in symptomatology for 6 months postoperatively, it is reasonable to be evaluated for surgical treatment of incontinence with a detailed history and physical, urinalysis and urine culture, ultrasound to determine post-void residual (PVR), cystoscopy, and urodynamics. Patients who demonstrate a significant sphincter defect and who report bothersome clinical symptoms should be referred for surgical treatment of postoperative incontinence. Some authors [15] suggest utilizing a validated questionnaire such as the International Consultation on Incontinence Questionnaire Short Form [27], the UCLA/RAND Prostate Cancer Index Urinary Function Score [28], the Patient's Global Impression of Improvement [29], or the Incontinence Impact Questionnaire Short Form [30] to help quantify the degree of bother and help stratify patients toward an appropriate treatment.

6.2 Traditional Open Approach to the Treatment of SUI Following Prostatectomy and Cystectomy (i.e., AUS)

Patients who are evaluated for surgical correction of postoperative incontinence have a number of possible surgical treatments. The artificial urinary sphincter (AUS) represents the gold standard treatment for moderate-severe urinary incontinence, prior failed AUS or sling procedures, patients with abnormal anatomy, or those with prior radiation or salvage treatment. Patients with previous radiation therapy followed by salvage treatment represent a particularly difficult patient population given high rates of incontinence in published studies following salvage treatment

[31] and should be treated with AUS given studies that have shown equivalent complication rates between patients who were treated with and without prior radiotherapy [32]. Additionally, patients with detrusor hypocontractility on pressure-flow urodynamics may not be able to generate enough force to overcome the fixed resistance of a compressive male sling and may be preferentially treated with AUS.

While the AUS represents an excellent surgical treatment for postoperative urinary incontinence, it does represent a fairly invasive and significant surgical intervention with potentially significant complications. Lai et al. [33] found that complications associated with AUS implantation included infection (5.5 %), erosion (6.0 %), mechanical failure (6.0 %), urethral atrophy (9.6 %), and surgical revision or removal (27.1 %) in a group of 270 patients undergoing AUS placement at a high-volume surgical center by a single surgeon.

An increasing body of literature has also identified the role of patient frailty and comorbidities in contributing toward postoperative surgical complications [34, 35]. For implantation of the AUS, prior studies have shown that increased comorbidities including hypertension, coronary artery disease, prior radiation treatment, and previous AUS revisions are at a higher risk for AUS cuff erosion [36]. While further research is necessary to identify how comorbidities impact AUS outcomes, patients with significant medical issues or less significant bother may benefit from a more minimally invasive approach to the treatment of their postsurgical urinary incontinence.

6.3 Minimally Invasive Approaches to Treating SUI Following Prostatectomy and Cystectomy

6.3.1 History

The management of urinary incontinence dates back in recorded history to the time of the Egyptians, with urinary incontinence being a known complication associated with spinal cord injuries, surgical intervention for bladder stones [37]. While the initial options for the treatment of urinary incontinence consisted of a variety of pharmacologic compounds or external devices designed to place pressure on the bulbar urethra, the first surgical treatment for postoperative urinary incontinence for a male was credited to Hugh Hampton Young who in 1907 performed a combined transvesical and perineal approach repair with exposure of the bladder mucosa, denuding the trigone and placating the bladder wall with deep sutures. While open surgical treatments for postoperative urinary incontinence have dramatically improved over the last 100 years, especially with the development of the gold standard treatment, the artificial urinary sphincter, a number of more minimally invasive treatments have been investigated.

6.3.2 Bulking Agents

A number of different urethral bulking agents or injection therapies have been evaluated as potential treatments for postoperative stress urinary incontinence.

Kuznetsov et al. [38] compared a cohort of patients treated with urethral collagen injection with a group that were treated with placement of an AUS. While this was not a true randomized trial given the difficulty in enrolling patients between two treatments with very different approaches and outcomes, at a mean follow-up of 19 months, the collagen group had a 20 % continence rate as compared to 75 % in the AUS group. Most available series have reported similarly limited efficacy, Smith et al. [39] reported social continence of 35.2 % following radical prostatectomy, while other series have been even more pessimistic, Griebling et al. [40] evaluated a series of 25 patients, of which only two patients (8 %) reported clinically significant improvement. Given the limited efficacy of most available evidence on bulking agent injections, submucosal injection of bulking agents is no longer part of the recommended treatment algorithm for postoperative urinary incontinence and has largely fallen out of favor with clinicians.

6.3.3   Male Slings

The male sling arose as a necessity to have a low-risk minimally invasive treatment for men with mild stress incontinence [41], which can be defined as a 24-h pad weight of less than 150 g [42]. They also can be utilized in patients with limited physical or cognitive capacity. The male sling imparts outlet resistance on the urethra without complete occlusion, thereby decreasing the risk of erosion and mechanical failure when compared to the AUS [43]. Berry [44] and Kaufman [45] described the first male slings, although these early models had low success rates and high complication rates. There are a range of contemporary male sling techniques that differ in their indications, rates of success, and complications [43]. Relative contraindications of slings include prior radiation therapy or urethral erosion, as their patients' incontinence typically exceeds the limits of the procedure [46]. Complications include perineal pain (usually resolves after 3 months but up to 74 % in bone-anchored system [46]), urinary retention (transient), infection, bone anchor complications (bone anchor system only), and rare erosion.

6.3.4   Bone-Anchored Bulbourethral Sling (InVance)

The InVance system (American Medical Systems) is a bone-anchored bulbourethral sling made of a 4 by 7 cm silicon-coated polymer. It is placed via a single perineal incision with dissection to the bulbospongiosus muscle and both ischiopubic rami – the sling is positioned under the bulbar urethra and fixed to the ischiopubic rami by three titanium screws bilaterally. The technique has short operative times, low erosion rate, and no need for retropubic passage of suspension sutures [47, 48]. The mechanism relies on compression of the urethra that results in a fixed increase in urethral resistance [49]. Determining the appropriate tension of the sling is the most critical portion of the operation: some utilize intraoperative measurement of the retrograde leak point pressure, with better outcomes from an RLPP greater than 60 cm over lower compression pressure [49], or an intraoperative cough test [47].

The results include pad-free rates ranging 36–85 % for patients with mild to severe incontinence [46, 50–54]. Common complications include transient perineal pain in up to 76 %, usually resolving 3 months postoperatively, increased residual urine (up to 12 %), infection leading to explanation (up to 15 %), and dislodgement from bone anchors (up to 5 %). InVance treatment failure is more common in men with previous history of irradiation [46, 54]. Other disadvantages include the high cost of bone screws and risk of osseous complications.

6.3.5   Transobturator Bulbourethral Sling (AdVance)

The AdVance sling (American Medical Systems) is a retrourethral transobturator sling which aims to restore the posterior urethra and sphincter region to the former preprostatectomy position [55]. Increased intraluminal resistance is achieved with a repositioned and lengthened membranous urethra [56]. In comparison to the InVance system, the AdVance system does not rely upon urethral compression, although some compression may place a role [57]. The system relies on good mobility of the sphincter region and good residual sphincter function including a coaptive zone of at least 1 cm [58]. Utilizing a perineal incision, polyprolene mesh is loosely positioned over the corpus spongiosum at the level of the perineal body, with the ends brought transobturator using a helical passing device. The mesh is tensioned to bring the perineal body and proximal bulbar urethra proximally and cephalad 2–4 cm, utilizing cystoscopic visualization of the external sphincter region to confirm the repositioning of the urethra. The sling functions "as a backstop" during straining [59].

Reported results with at least 1-year follow-up include up to 70 % dry rates [55, 58, 60–64] and 25–53 % dry rates in patients with previous irradiation [61, 63, 65]. Rehder et al. [66] reported 76.8 % success rate at 3 years with proper sling fixation, although a Cleveland Clinic report noted a decline in patient-determined success from 87.3 to 62.5 % at 2 years postoperatively [67]. Complications include transient acute postoperative urinary retention requiring catheterization (up to 21 %), wound infection, urinary tract infection, or persistent perineal pain. In addition, the need for explantation is much lower than InVance system. In the case of a failed AdVance sling with good sphincter function, a second sling can be implanted, as Soljanik et al. [68] describe, with results showing 34.5 % of patients with no pad use, 38 % with one dry "security" pad use.

6.3.6   Prepubic and Transobturator Sling (Virtue)

The Virtue quadratic sling (Coloplast, Denmark) is a hybrid device (four-armed large pore knitted monofilament polyprolene mesh) that provides proximal urethral relocation with a transobturator component and perineal compression with a superior prepubic component [70]. The sling is placed via a perineal incision with dissection exposing the bulbous urethra and pubic rami, detaching the urethra from the perineal body but leaving the bulbospongiosus muscle intact. The sling's two lateral extensions are bilaterally pulled transobturator via a curved introducer inserted through the ipsilateral groin crease just inferior to the adductor longus tendon. The sling's two superior extensions are bilaterally pulled superior and anterior to the pubic bone via a curved introducer. The transobturator extensions are pulled laterally until the bulbar urethra moves 2–3 cm proximally. The superior extensions are pulled superiorly to provide visual compression of the bulbar and perineal urethra, adjusting the tension to increase the retrograde leak point pressure to 60–70 cm water.

The results of the Virtue system trial at 1 year postoperatively showed 42 % of subjects with >50 % reduction in mean pad weight [69]. There was a decline in efficacy over the first 12 months postoperatively, from initial 61 % >50 % reduction in mean pad weight at 1.5 months down to 42 % at 12 months.

Comiter et al. also attempted "sling fixation," enrolling a cohort of 21 patients 12 months after Virtue placement [69]. Virtue fixation consists of subcutaneously tunneling the transobturator extensions medially and suturing them together and suturing the superior extensions in a figure of eight under tension verified by RLPP. The Virtue system with fixation improved the continence result and showed 79 % of subjects with >50 % reduction in mean pad weight at 1 year postoperatively [69].

Advantages of this system include utilizing two commentary mechanisms to increase intraluminal urethral pressure. The prepubic component fixes the system in place and prevents proximal sling migration, which can be a cause of retroluminal sling failure [70–72]. The prepubic provides urethral compression without bone screws, which eliminates the risk of anchor-associated osseous complications.

6.3.7 Suburethral Sling (Remeex)

The Remeex system (Neomedic, Spain) is a readjustable sling positioned underneath the bulbar urethra, consisting of a mesh connected via two monofilament traction threads to an implanted suprapubic mechanical regulator implanted subcutaneously over the rectus fascia 2 cm superior to the pubis. An external manipulator can adjust the device. Sousa-Escandon et al. [73] reported dry rate of 83 % at mean 18 months, Campos-Fernandes et al. [74] reported dry rate of 55.5 % at mean 26.3 months, and Sousa-Escandon et al. [75] reported dry rate of 64.7 % at mean 32 months. The majority of patients require at least one adjustment to reach maximum benefit. Complications include intraoperative bladder injuries (up to 11 %) and rate of up to 12 % device explantation secondary to urethral erosion or infection. The system has high reported rate of perineal pain.

6.3.8 Argus Sling

The Argus system (Promedon, Argentina) consists of retrobulbar placement of a radiopaque silicon foam pad for soft compression of the bulbar urethra, with two attached silicon columns consisting of multiple conical elements that allow for system readjustment. These two columns track anteriorly to two fixed radiopaque silicon washers which regulate the desired tension. The sling is sequentially adjusted to achieve a final resting leak point pressure of between 20 and 48 cm water prior to closure of the incision. The device can be implanted either retropubic or transobturator. Romano et al. [76] reported 66% dry rate at mean 45-month follow-up with 10.4% readjustment, and Hubner et al. [77] reported 79.2% dry rate at mean 50.4 months with 28.6% readjustment. Complications include 15% transient perineal pain and 8–12% sling explantation due to erosion into the urethra and bladder through the abdominal wall or due to infection.

6.3.9   Prostate Adjustable Continence Therapy Device (ProACT)

The adjustable continence therapy device (ProACT*TM* Uromedica, Plymouth, MN, USA) is a treatment device which consists of two balloons which are placed bilaterally along the urethra at the bladder neck via a perineal approach under fluoroscopic guidance with a cystoscope sheath inserted in the bladder to serve as a guide for placement. The tubing and port of the ProACT systems are placed in the scrotum which is an advantage over many other treatments of post prostatectomy incontinence in that the balloons are accessible and can be adjusted after placement depending on patient symptomatology. Hübner and Schlarp published a prospective series of 117 consecutive men who underwent ProACT with a mean follow-up of 13 months with an overall 67% rate of patients reporting total continence and 92% reporting significant improvement [78]. Reoperation rates of 27% ($n=32$) in this study were similar to those reported for large AUS series, and similar to the 17–30% reported in other large series [79–81]. One advantage of the adjustable continence therapy device is the ability to modulate the amount of compression as patients who experienced postoperative urinary retention could be treated with withdrawal of a small amount of fluid from the coapting balloons. Patients should be counseled preoperatively that balloon adjustments may be a critical component of this treatment. For the large available series on the implantation of the ProACT system, almost all patients required some adjustment, the average number of adjustments varied from 3 to 4.6 [78, 79, 81] with a mean balloon volume of 3.1–3.8 ml [78–80]. Another is the relatively short operative time needed to place the system, as mean operative times for the placement of ProACT in experienced center have been reported as between 18 and 37 min [80, 82]. In order to better assess reoperation rates compared to their prior study which included their initial implantations, Hübner and Schlarp published a follow-up study [83] that compared their first 50 cases demonstrating much lower rates of complications requiring revision surgery (24% as compared to 58%) for patients treated following the initial learning curve. More recently, some clinicians have utilized a modified transrectal ultrasound (TRUS)-guided placement of the ProACT in an attempt to limit the radiation exposure with the traditional fluoroscopic placement. Gregori et al. [84] reported their results with this technique for 79 patients reporting a 66.1% dry rate (as defined as a 24-h pad test with <8 g leakage) and a mean of 3.6 adjustments per patient, similar rates to the fluoroscopically inserted series with lower rates of erosion (3.2%) and device migration (4.8%) for long-term complications.

6.4   Future Directions and Conclusions

One intriguing frontier in the treatment of urinary incontinence is the use of periurethral injections of adipose-derived regenerative cells or stem cells. Yamamoto et al. [85] evaluated the effect regenerative cells which were transurethrally injected into the rhabdosphincter and submucosal space of the urethra in a small case series of three patients noting a progressive improvement in urinary symptoms in terms of decreased leakage volume, decreased frequency, decreased amount of incontinence, and improved quality of life. Post-injection MRI imaging suggested persistence of injected adipose tissue. The 1-year follow-up data by this group on 11 patients injected with the same technique demonstrated similar improvement in urinary symptoms as well as improved mean maximum urethral closing pressure and functional profile length of the sphincter [86]. As these studies have been small clinical trials without a control arm, it is unclear if the improvements noted in symptomatology represent a normal improvement incontinence following prostatectomy. This treatment remains an experimental option for the treatment of incontinence and is not currently recommended in guidelines for the treatment of post-prostatectomy incontinence [15]. However, injection of regenerative stem cells remains a novel treatment option that may prove beneficial with further validation.

The minimally invasive treatment of postsurgical incontinence represents an area of tremendous potential for innovation and improvement. One persistent issue with the available evidence on minimally invasive treatments for incontinence following surgery is the reliance on single institution and often single-surgeon studies. While control groups and the creation of randomized control trials are often difficult or ethically impossible, care should be taken in future studies to incorporate multiple high-volume institutions and surgeons in collaborative studies, pursue more robust follow-up periods, and use standardized and validated metrics for measuring quality of life and urinary incontinence symptoms to better assess the efficacy and durability of these techniques. This standardization would allow for greater generalizability and a higher quality of available data on these emerging minimally invasive approaches.

Stress urinary incontinence represents a significant and common complication following urological surgery with a significant impact on patient quality of life, and the development of effective, minimally invasive treatments represents an important clinical goal. A number of available treatments including male slings and the prostate adjustable continence device provide reliable outcomes and improved quality of life for patients with persistent postsurgical incontinence, while experimental treatments may provide further options for patients with this common complication following urological surgery.

References

1. de Moor JS, Mariotto AB, Parry C, et al. Cancer survivors in the United States: prevalence across the survivorship trajectory and implications for care. Cancer Epidemiol Biomarkers Prev. 2013;22:561.

2. Cooperberg MR, Broering JM, Carroll PR. Time trends and local variation in primary treatment of localized prostate cancer. J Clin Oncol. 2010;28:1117.

3. Foote J, Yun S, Leach GE. Postprostatectomy incontinence. Pathophysiology, evaluation, and management. Urol Clin N Am. 1991;18:229.

4. Coelho RF, Rocco B, Patel MB, et al. Retropubic, laparoscopic, and robot-assisted radical prostatectomy: a critical review of outcomes reported by high-volume centers. J Endourol. 2010;24:2003.

5. Ficarra V, Novara G, Fracalanza S, et al. A prospective, non-randomized trial comparing robot-assisted laparoscopic and retropubic radical prostatectomy in one European institution. BJU Int. 2009;104:534.

6. Ficarra V, Novara G, Rosen RC, et al. Systematic review and meta-analysis of studies reporting urinary continence recovery after robot-assisted radical prostatectomy. Eur Urol. 2012;62:405.

7. Carlsson S, Nilsson AE, Schumacher MC, et al. Surgery-related complications in 1253 robot-assisted and 485 open retropubic radical prostatectomies at the Karolinska University Hospital, Sweden. Urology. 2010;75:1092.

8. Dobbs RW, Kocjancic E, Crivellaro S. Male stress urinary incontinence following surgical intervention: procedures, technical modifications, and patient considerations. In: Del Popolo G, Pistolesi D, Li Marzi V, editors. Male stress urinary incontinence. Cham, Switzerland: Springer International Publishing; 2015. p. 45–72.

9. Glickman L, Godoy G, Lepor H. Changes in continence and erectile function between 2 and 4 years after radical prostatectomy. J Urol. 2009;181:731.

10. Hautmann RE, Sauter TW, Wenderoth UK. Radical retropubic prostatectomy: morbidity and urinary continence in 418 consecutive cases. Urology. 1994;43:47.

11. Wei JT, Dunn RL, Marcovich R, et al. Prospective assessment of patient reported urinary continence after radical prostatectomy. J Urol. 2000;164:744.

12. Van Kampen M, De Weerdt W, Van Poppel H, et al. Effect of pelvic-floor re-education on duration and degree of incontinence after radical prostatectomy: a randomised controlled trial. Lancet. 2000;355:98.

13. Filocamo MT, Li Marzi V, Del Popolo G, et al. Effectiveness of early pelvic floor rehabilitation treatment for post-prostatectomy incontinence. Eur Urol. 2005;48:734.

14. Goode PS, Burgio KL, Johnson 2nd TM, et al. Behavioral therapy with or without biofeedback and pelvic floor electrical stimulation for persistent postprostatectomy incontinence: a randomized controlled trial. JAMA. 2011;305:151.

15. Bauer RM, Gozzi C, Hubner W, et al. Contemporary management of postprostatectomy incontinence. Eur Urol. 2011;59:985.

16. Penson DF, McLerran D, Feng Z, et al. 5-year urinary and sexual outcomes after radical prostatectomy: results from the prostate cancer outcomes study. J Urol. 2005;173:1701.

17. Prabhu V, Sivarajan G, Taksler GB, et al. Long-term continence outcomes in men undergoing radical prostatectomy for clinically localized prostate cancer. Eur Urol. 2014;65:52.

18. Thuroff JW, Mattiasson A, Andersen JT, et al. The standardization of terminology and assessment of functional characteristics of intestinal urinary reservoirs. Scand J Urol Nephrol. 1996;30:349.

19. Steers WD. Voiding dysfunction in the orthotopic neobladder. World J Urol. 2000;18:330.

20. Kessler TM, Burkhard FC, Perimenis P, et al. Attempted nerve sparing surgery and age have a significant effect on urinary continence and erectile function after radical cystoprostatectomy and ileal orthotopic bladder substitution. J Urol. 2004;172:1323–7.

21. El Bahnasawy MS, Osman Y, Gomha MA, et al. Nocturnal enuresis in men with an orthotopic ileal reservoir: urodynamic evaluation. J Urol. 2000;164:10.

22. Elmajian DA, Stein JP, Esrig D, et al. The Kock ileal neobladder: updated experience in 295 male patients. J Urol. 1996;156:920.

23. Granberg CF, Boorjian SA, Crispen PL, et al. Functional and oncological outcomes after orthotopic neobladder reconstruction in women. BJU Int. 2008;102:1551–5.

24. Grossfeld GD, Stein JP, Bennett J, et al. Lower urinary tract reconstruction in the female using the Kock ileal reservoir with bilateral ureteroileal urethrostomy: update of continence results and fluorourodynamic findings. Urology. 1996;48:383–8.

25. Parekh AR, Feng MI, Kirages D, et al. The role of pelvic floor exercises on post-prostatectomy incontinence. J Urol. 2003;170:130–3.
26. Skinner EC MD, Skinner DG MD, Stein JP MD, Orthotopic Urinary Diversion. Campbell-Walsh urology. 10th ed. Philadelphia: Elsevier-Saunders; 2012. p. 2479–506. Chapter 87.
27. Avery K, Donovan J, Peters TJ, et al. ICIQ: a brief and robust measure for evaluating the symptoms and impact of urinary incontinence. Neurourol Urodyn. 2004;23:322.
28. Litwin MS, Hays RD, Fink A, et al. The UCLA prostate cancer index: development, reliability, and validity of a health-related quality of life measure. Med Care. 1998;36:1002.
29. Yalcin I, Bump RC. Validation of two global impression questionnaires for incontinence. Am J Obstet Gynecol. 2003;189:98.
30. Uebersax JS, Wyman JF, Shumaker SA, et al. Short forms to assess life quality and symptom distress for urinary incontinence in women: the incontinence impact questionnaire and the urogenital distress inventory. Continence program for women research group. Neurourol Urodyn. 1995;14:131.
31. Marcus DM, Canter DJ, Jani AB, et al. Salvage therapy for locally recurrent prostate cancer after radiation. Can J Urol. 2012;19:6534.
32. Gomha MA, Boone TB. Artificial urinary sphincter for post-prostatectomy incontinence in men who had prior radiotherapy: a risk and outcome analysis. J Urol. 2002;167:591.
33. Lai HH, Hsu EI, Teh BS, et al. 13 years of experience with artificial urinary sphincter implantation at Baylor College of Medicine. J Urol. 2007;177:1021.
34. Revenig LM, Canter DJ, Taylor MD, et al. Too frail for surgery? Initial results of a large multidisciplinary prospective study examining preoperative variables predictive of poor surgical outcomes. J Am Coll Surg. 2013;217:665.
35. Revenig LM, Canter DJ, Master VA, et al. A prospective study examining the association between preoperative frailty and postoperative complications in patients undergoing minimally invasive surgery. J Endourol. 2014;28:476.
36. Raj GV, Peterson AC, Webster GD. Outcomes following erosions of the artificial urinary sphincter. J Urol. 2006;175:2186.
37. Schultheiss D, Hofner K, Oelke M, et al. Historical aspects of the treatment of urinary incontinence. Eur Urol. 2000;38:352.
38. Kuznetsov DD, Kim HL, Patel RV, et al. Comparison of artificial urinary sphincter and collagen for the treatment of postprostatectomy incontinence. Urology. 2000;56:600.
39. Smith DN, Appell RA, Rackley RR, et al. Collagen injection therapy for post-prostatectomy incontinence. J Urol. 1998;160:364.
40. Griebling TL, Kreder Jr KJ, Williams RD. Transurethral collagen injection for treatment of postprostatectomy urinary incontinence in men. Urology. 1997;49:907.
41. Kumar A, Litt ER, Ballert KN, Nitti VW. Artificial urinary sphincter versus male sling for post-prostatectomy incontinence—what do patients choose? J Urol. 2009;181:1231–5.
42. Flynn BJ, Webster GD. Evaluation and surgical management of intrinsic sphincter deficiency after radical prostatectomy. Rev Urol. 2004;6:180–6.
43. Comiter CV. Surgery insight: surgical management of postprostatectomy incontinence-the artificial urinary sphincter and male sling. Nat Clin Pract Urol. 2007;4:615–24.
44. Berry J. New procedure for correction of urinary incontinence: a preliminary report. J Urol. 1961;85:771–5.
45. Kaufman JJ. Urethral compression operations for the treatment of post-prostatectomy incontinence. J Urol. 1973;110:93–6.
46. Giberti C, Gallo F, Schenone M, Cortese P, Ninotta G. The bone anchor suburethral synthetic sling for iatrogenic male incontinence: critical evaluation at a mean 3-year followup. J Urol. 2009;181:2204–8.
47. Madjar S, Jacoby K, Giberti C, et al. Bone anchored sling for the treatment of post-prostatectomy incontinence. J Urol. 2001;165:72–6.
48. Comiter CV. The male sling for stress urinary incontinence: a prospective study. J Urol. 2002;167:597–601.
49. Ullrich NF, Comiter CV. The male sling for stress urinary incontinence: urodynamic and subjective assessment. J Urol. 2004;172:204–6.

50. Comiter CV. The male perineal sling: intermediate-term results. Neurourol Urodyn. 2005;24: 648–53.
51. Fassi-Fehri H, Badet L, Cherass A, et al. Efficacy of the InVance™ male sling in men with stress urinary incontinence. Eur Urol. 2007;51:498–503.
52. Giberti C, Gallo F, Schenone M, Cortese P. The bone-anchor sub- urethral sling for the treatment of iatrogenic male incontinence: subjective and objective assessment after 41 months of mean follow-up. World J Urol. 2008;26:173–8.
53. Guimaraes M, Oliveira R, Pinto R, et al. Intermediate-term results, up to 4 years, of a bone-anchored male perineal sling for treating male stress urinary incontinence after prostate surgery. BJU Int. 2009;103:500–4.
54. Carmel M, Hage B, Hanna S, Schmutz G, Tu LM. Long-term efficacy of the bone-anchored male sling for moderate and severe stress urinary incontinence. BJU Int. 2010;106:1012–6.
55. Rehder P, Gozzi C. Transobturator sling suspension for male urinary incontinence including post-radical prostatectomy. Eur Urol. 2007;52:860–7.
56. Firrozi F, Vasavada S. Editorial comment. Urodynamic changes and initial results of the AdVance male sling. Urology. 2009;74:357–8.
57. Latini JM. Editorial comment. Urodynamic changes and initial results of the AdVance male sling. Urology. 2009;74:358.
58. Rehder P, Freiin von Gleissenthall G, Pichler R, Glodny B. The treatment of postprostatectomy incontinence with the retroluminal transobturator repositioning sling (advance1): lessons learnt from accumulative experience. Arch Esp Urol. 2009;62:860–70.
59. De Ridder D, Rehder P. The advance male sling: anatomic features in relation to mode of action. Eur Urol Suppl. 2011;10:383–9.
60. Bauer RM, Mayer ME, Gratzke C, et al. Prospective evaluation of the functional sling suspension for male postprostatectomy stress urinary incontinence: results after 1 year. Eur Urol. 2009;56:928–33.
61. Cornu J-N, Se' be P, Ciofu C, et al. The advance transobturator male sling for post prostatectomy incontinence: clinical results of a prospective evaluation after a minimum follow-up of 6 months. Eur Urol. 2009;56:923–7.
62. Cornel EB, Elzevier HW, Putter H. Can advance transobturator sling suspension cure male urinary postoperative stress incontinence? J Urol. 2010;183:1459–63.
63. Cornu JN, Sebe P, Ciofu C, Peyrat L, Cussenot O, Haab F. Mid-term evaluation of the transobturator male sling for post-prostatectomy incontinence: focus on prognostic factors. BJU Int. 2011;108:236–40.
64. Bauer RM, Soljanik I, Füllhase C, et al. Mid-term results of the retroluminar transobturator sling suspension for male postprostatectomy stress urinary incontinence. BJU Int. 2011;108:94–8.
65. Bauer RM, Soljanik I, Fu¨llhase C, et al. Results of the advance transobturator male sling after radical prostatectomy and adjuvant radiotherapy. Urology. 2011;77:474–9.
66. Rehder P, Haab F, Cornu JN, et al. Treatment of post prostatectomy male urinary incontinence with the transobturator retroluminal repositioning sling suspension: 3year followup. Eur Urol. 2012;62:140–5.
67. Li H, Gill BC, Nowacki AS, et al. Therapeutic durability of the male transobturator sling: midterm patient reported outcomes. J Urol. 2012;187:1331–5.
68. Soljanik I, Becker AJ, Stief CG, Gozzi C, Bauer RM. Repeat retro- urethral transobturator sling in the management of recurrent post prostatectomy stress urinary incontinence after failed first male sling. Eur Urol. 2010;58:767–72.
69. Comiter CV, Rhee EY, Tu LM, Herschorn S, Nitti VW. The virtue sling – a new quadratic sling for post prostatectomy incontinence – results of a multinational clinical trial. Urology. 2014;84(2):433–8. doi:10.1016/j.urology.2014.02.062. Epub 2014 Jun 25.
70. Comiter CV, Nitti V, Elliott C, Rhee E. A new quadratic sling for male stress incontinence: retrograde leak point pressure as a measure of urethral resistance. J Urol. 2012;187:563–8.
71. Yiou R, Loche CM, Lingombet O, et al. Evaluation of urinary symptoms in patients with postprostatectomy urinary incontinence treated with the male sling TOMS. Neurourol Urodyn. 2015;34:12–7.

72. Fisher MB, Aggarwal N, Vuruskan H, Singla AK. Efficacy of artificial urinary sphincter implantation after failed bone-anchored male sling for post prostatectomy incontinence. Urology. 2007;70:942–4.
73. Sousa-Escandon A, Rodriguez Gomez JI, Uribarri Gonzalez C, Marques-Queimadelos A. Externally readjustable sling for treatment of male stress urinary incontinence: points of technique and preliminary results. J Endourol. 2004;18:113–8.
74. Campos-Fernandes JL, Timsit MO, Paparel P, et al. REMEEX: a possible treatment option in selected cases of sphincter incompetence [in French]. Prog Urol. 2006;16:184–91.
75. Sousa-Escandon A, Cabrera J, Mantovani F, et al. Adjustable suburethral sling (male Remeex system1) in the treatment of male stress urinary incontinence: a multicentric European study. Eur Urol. 2007;52:1473–80.
76. Romano SV, Metrebian SE, Vaz F, et al. Long-term results of a phase III multicentre trial of the adjustable male sling for treating urinary incontinence after prostatectomy: minimum 3 years [in Spanish]. Actas Urol Esp. 2009;33:309–14.
77. Hubner WA, Gallistl H, Rutkowski M, Huber ER. Adjustable bulbourethral male sling: experience after 101 cases of moderate-to-severe male stress urinary incontinence. BJU Int. 2011; 107:777–82.
78. Hubner WA, Schlarp OM. Treatment of incontinence after prostatectomy using a new minimally invasive device: adjustable continence therapy. BJU Int. 2005;96:587.
79. Kocjancic E, Crivellaro S, Ranzoni S, et al. Adjustable continence therapy for the treatment of male stress urinary incontinence: a single-centre study. Scand J Urol Nephrol. 2007;41:324.
80. Lebret T, Cour F, Benchetrit J, et al. Treatment of post prostatectomy stress urinary incontinence using a minimally invasive adjustable continence balloon device, ProACT: results of a preliminary, multicenter, pilot study. Urology. 2008;71:256.
81. Trigo-Rocha F, Gomes CM, Pompeo AC, et al. Prospective study evaluating efficacy and safety of Adjustable Continence Therapy (ProACT) for post radical prostatectomy urinary incontinence. Urology. 2006;67:965.
82. Crivellaro S, Singla A, Aggarwal N, et al. Adjustable continence therapy (ProACT) and bone anchored male sling: comparison of two new treatments of post prostatectomy incontinence. Int J Urol. 2008;15:910.
83. Hubner WA, Schlarp OM. Adjustable continence therapy (ProACT): evolution of the surgical technique and comparison of the original 50 patients with the most recent 50 patients at a single centre. Eur Urol. 2007;52:680.
84. Gregori A, Romano AL, Scieri F, et al. Transrectal ultrasound-guided implantation of Adjustable Continence Therapy (ProACT): surgical technique and clinical results after a mean follow-up of 2 years. Eur Urol. 2010;57:430.
85. Yamamoto T, Gotoh M, Kato M, et al. Periurethral injection of autologous adipose-derived regenerative cells for the treatment of male stress urinary incontinence: report of three initial cases. Int J Urol. 2012;19:652.
86. Gotoh M, Yamamoto T, Kato M, et al. Regenerative treatment of male stress urinary incontinence by periurethral injection of autologous adipose-derived regenerative cells: 1-year outcomes in 11 patients. Int J Urol. 2014;21:294.

Preserving Sexual Function and Continence during Radical Hysterectomy

Fabio Landoni, Vanna Zanagnolo, and Marco Soligo

7.1   Introduction

Cervical cancer is, after breast cancer, the second highest worldwide female malignancy. The incidence has been increasing gradually over recent years, with younger patients resulting affected. Thus, it is becoming one of the most deadly cancer globally [1–4].

The age-adjusted incidence rate rises rapidly in the third decade of life to approximately 20 cases per 100,000 and then increases slowly to 30 through the ninth decade. Although cervical cytology may potentially reduce the mortality rate of cervical cancer by 80 %, this procedure has only been fully implemented in few countries because of its costs and logistical problems resulting from the high incidence of cervical cancer precursors [5].

Various types of radical surgery (RS), such as radical hysterectomy, radical trachelectomy, and radical parametrectomy, have shown 5-year survival rates ranging between 75 and 90 % [1, 5, 6], remaining the standard treatment for patients with early-stage cervical cancer [7–9]. However, RS is known to cause urinary dysfunctions, such as bladder hypotonia, urinary incontinence, and abnormal sensation, in 12–85 % of patients [10–12]. Furthermore, bowel dysfunctions, such as constipation, have been reported in 5–10 % of patients after RS [13, 14].

Considerable sexual dysfunctions, including decrease in sexual interest, orgasm, and vaginal dryness, may also be reported after RS. The sexual activity impairment thus results in substantial distress [15]. Urinary, anorectal, and sexual dysfunctions are known to be caused, during RS, by the disruption of sympathetic and parasympathetic

F. Landoni • V. Zanagnolo
Gynecology Department IEO, European Institute Oncology, Milan, Italy

M. Soligo (✉)
Obstetrics and Gynecology Department, Vittore Buzzi Hospital, ICP, Milan, Italy
e-mail: marcosoligo@fastwebnet.it

© Springer International Publishing Switzerland 2016
A. Carbone et al. (eds.), *Functional Urologic Surgery in Neurogenic and Oncologic Diseases*, Urodynamics, Neurourology and Pelvic Floor Dysfunctions, DOI 10.1007/978-3-319-29191-8_7

nerves that are intimately associated with the supporting tissues of the cervix, bladder, and rectum, i.e., the paracervix (cardinal ligaments), the rectal stalk (lateral ligament of the rectum), the vesicouterine ligaments (lateral leaf), and the uterosacral ligaments. These nerves play a major role in the neurogenic control of urinary and anorectal functions. Moreover, they supply blood vessels of the female genital tract and thereby affect sexual activity by neurogenically controlling its lubrication or swelling response [16].

7.2　Relevant Pelvic Floor Neuroanatomy and Physiology

The pelvic floor is under autonomic (sympathetic and parasympathetic) and somatic control.

The sympathetic fibers innervating the pelvis arise from the para-aortic sympathetic chain at the T11–L2 level. These fibers synapse in the superior hypogastric plexus and course into the pelvis over the sacral promontory. They enter the pelvis via the hypogastric nerve and synapse in the pelvic plexus (inferior hypogastric plexus). In the pelvic plexus, those fibers synapse with parasympathetic fibers from S2 to S4, which traverse the pelvis via the pelvic nerve and enter the pelvic plexus from either side of the rectum. The postganglionic fibers may be exclusively sympathetic, exclusively parasympathetic, or a combination of both. At the points of junction of these nerves, small ganglia are found. From these plexuses, numerous branches accompany the collaterals of the hypogastric artery and are distributed to the rectum, cervix, lateral vagina, and bladder. Noteworthy, the pelvic plexus gives rise to postganglionic fibers which lie, as a flat meshed band, on the lateral wall of the upper third of the vagina. These fibers reach the bladder through the deep layer of the cervico-vesical and the vagino-vesical ligaments [17, 18].

7.2.1　Urinary Continence Control

During the *storage phase*, the bladder and the internal urethral sphincter are primarily under sympathetic nervous system control. Sympathetic nervous mediators activate β-adrenergic receptors within the bladder: this results in relaxation, promoting the bladder to increase its capacity without increasing detrusor resting pressure (accommodation). The same sympathetic mediators act on the bladder neck and internal urinary sphincter via α-adrenergic receptors to remain tightly closed. Finally, this sympathetic activity also inhibits parasympathetic stimulation via a feedback mechanism running through the spine to the encephalic pontine micturition center (PMC). On the other hand, the parasympathetic nervous system functions in an opposite manner. In terms of urinary function, it stimulates the detrusor to contract via acetylcholine activation of muscarinic receptors. When the sympathetic nervous system is active, urinary accommodation occurs and the micturition reflex is inhibited.

During the *voiding phase*, clearly a mechanism under voluntary control, the activity of the somatic component of the pudendal nerve is inhibited to cause the levator ani muscles to relax and the external urethral sphincter to open. Immediately preceding parasympathetic stimulation, the sympathetic influence on the internal urethral sphincter is suppressed allowing the bladder neck and the internal sphincter to relax and open. This results in the facilitation of voluntary urination.

Bladder and urethral sensation is of paramount importance to coordinate the aforementioned mechanism. Sensation within the bladder is transmitted to the central nervous system through sensory afferent fibers of the autonomic pathway. Urethral smooth and striated muscle afferent nerve fibers travel in the pudendal nerve and terminate at the dorsal sacral cord, S2–S4 [17, 19].

7.2.2 Anorectal Continence Control

Adequate bowel function is a rather complex phenomena resulting from a combination of stool consistency, colorectal activity, and the relationship between the internal anal sphincter (IAS) and external anal sphincter (EAS). The nerve supplying the rectum and anal canal derives from the superior, middle, and inferior rectal plexus with a relevant component of autonomic nerve fibers headed to the rectum and IAS coming from the inferior hypogastric plexus.

Similarly to what happens in urinary control, stimulation of parasympathetic nerves in the rectum encourages contraction of the reservoir (the rectum), while efferent rectal sympathetic fibers are thought to inhibit rectal contraction and stimulate the IAS contraction [20]. As a general rule, the anal continence mechanism implies a strict coordination between the sensory component and the reflex and voluntary (respectively, autonomic and somatic) control of the sphincter complex: the IAS maintains a constant tone and prevents fecal leakage, with the EAS and pelvic floor muscles acting as an additional barrier to prevent inappropriate defecation.

The sensory component is relevant here. The pectinate line within the cranial portion of the anal canal has the peculiar role to discriminate bowel content. When the bolus distends the ano-rectum, the rectoanal inhibitory reflex (RAIR) occurs: a transient reflex inhibition of the IAS tone to allow the bowel content to come in contact with the pectinate line and concomitant reflex contraction of the EAS to maintain continence for a limited time. The RAIR acts as a sampling reflex. If defecation is inappropriate, voluntary pelvic floor muscles and EAS contraction can push up the bowel content abolishing the reflex stimulation. On the contrary, pelvic floor muscles and EAS relaxation will promote sympathetic inhibition and parasympathetic activation with IAS relaxation and rectal detrusor activation [21].

7.3 Pathophysiology of Pelvic Floor Dysfunctions (PFDs) after Radical Surgery (RS) and Rationale for Nerve-Sparing Radical Surgery (NSRS)

During RS the hypogastric nerves and both the proximal and distal part of the inferior hypogastric plexus are routinely damaged.

PFDs are caused by neural denervation in combination with potential direct visceral injury, lymph stasis, interruption of the blood supply, and fibrosis. Moreover, particularly for the lower urinary tract, a substantial alteration of sensation for bladder filling is an additional evidence of pelvic sympathetic trunk injury.

The loss of sympathetic adrenergic stimulation may have an excitatory effect on parasympathetic transmission to the detrusor muscle during urine storage and may lead to permanent relaxation of the bladder neck and the proximal urethra. These alterations could contribute to the characterization of urinary stress incontinence and detrusor overactivity after RS [18].

The extent of neural damage is associated with more severe PFDs.

To reduce postoperative complications, it has been suggested to tailor the radicality of RH; however, such an aim could inevitably decrease operation efficacy [22]. Therefore, it has also been suggested to preserve the pelvic splanchnic nerves (PSN) without compromising the therapeutic effect of radical surgery.

Thus, NSRS has emerged in the last 30 years in order to reduce surgery-related dysfunctions without compromising oncologic outcomes [23, 24]. Not only is NSRH of great clinical interest in gynecologic oncology treatment for preserving the therapeutic effect but also for effectively improving the quality of life of patients [25].

7.4 Radical Hysterectomy

In 2007 a conference of international experts was convened in Kyoto, Japan, to discuss a new classification for RH. There has been a growing dissatisfaction with the Rutledge class II (type II; modified) and class III (type III) designation because the common practice no longer adheres to the original published descriptions *by Piver* [26]. This is also true when surgeons refer to an eponymous RH such as a Wertheim, or Meigs, or Okabayashi. In fact, procedures seldom conform to the original published descriptions. Furthermore, a number of important developments in the technique of RH are not considered by these classification systems, such as the various nerve-sparing dissections, fertility-preserving operations, and variations not fitting the Rutledge class II or class III category.

A proposal for a uniform anatomic terminology and a classification of RH and lymphadenectomy incorporating the opinions expressed by experts during the conference was published by *Querleu and Morrow* in 2008 [27].

As already mentioned, tailoring has become a major issue in cancer surgery. Modulation of radicality to tumor spread is an important topic in cervical cancer, based on the concept of the surgical margins and on the estimated risk of pericervical spread, from the development of ultraradical surgery to more limited types (i.e., modified radical) of it [27].

7.4.1 Querleu and Morrow Classification [27]

7.4.1.1 Type A: Minimum Resection of Paracervix

This resection is an extrafascial hysterectomy, with no need to free the ureters from their beds. The paracervix is transected medial to the ureter but lateral to the cervix.

The uterosacral and vesicouterine ligaments are not transected at a distance from the uterus.

7.4.1.2 Type B: Transection of Paracervix at the Ureter

Partial resection of the uterosacral and vesicouterine ligaments are standard steps of this type of radical hysterectomy. The ureter is unroofed and then rolled laterally to enable transection of the paracervix at the level of the ureteral tunnel. The posterior, deep, neural component of the paracervix, caudal to the deep uterine vein, is not resected. At least 10 mm of the vagina from the cervix is removed.

7.4.1.3 Type C: Transection of Paracervix at Junction with Internal Iliac Vascular System

This type of radical hysterectomy encompasses transection of the uterosacral ligament at the rectum and vesicouterine ligament at the bladder. The ureter is mobilized completely. Fifteen to 20 mm of vagina from the cervix with the adjacent paracolpos are resected as well.

Two subcategories are defined: *C1 with nerve preservation* and *C2*, without preservation of autonomic nerves. In C1, the sacrouterine ligament is transected after separation of the hypogastric nerves. The nerve is identified systematically and preserved by transection of only the uterine branches of the pelvic plexus. The bladder branches of the pelvic plexus are preserved in the lateral ligament of the bladder (i.e., lateral part of bladder pillar). When the caudal part of the paracervix is transected, careful identification of bladder nerves is needed. For C2, the paracervix is transected completely, including the part caudal to the deep uterine vein.

7.4.1.4 Type D: Laterally Extended Resection

This group of rare operations feature additional ultraradical procedures, mostly indicated at the time of pelvic exenteration.

7.4.2 Concept of Nerve-Sparing Surgery [5]

Radical hysterectomy is meant to remove the tissue adjacent to the cervix and vaginal fornices in addition to the uterus, cervix, and proximal vagina, preserving intact both the urinary system and rectum. The removal of the surrounding tissues of the cervix and adjacent vagina is necessary because they are the first to be invaded by contiguity and local lymphatic extension of cervical cancer. The major difficulty to perform this operation is that the ureters pass through the paracervix and paracolpos and therefore must be carefully dissected off to prevent injury.

Over the last decade, many studies have been published in the literature on the topic of nerve-sparing RH, reporting outcomes and describing various techniques, sometimes with emphasis on the hypogastric nerves, the pelvic splanchnic nerves, or the bladder branches of the IHP [25, 28–37].

Some variations of RH are by default "nerve sparing," such as the simple, intra- or extrafascial hysterectomy, Rutledge class II, types A and B RH of the new classification in which the autonomic nerve supply to the bladder is not threatened.

However, more radical removal of the supporting tissues of the cervix requires special surgical maneuvers to preserve the autonomic nerves associated with the uterosacral ligaments, vesicouterine ligaments, and the paracervix as it is described in *Type C1* nerve-sparing RH.

The main steps essential of the nerve-sparing radical hysterectomy (NSRH) are:

1. Identification of the hypogastric nerve in the mesoureter and separation of the mesoureter and the hypogastric nerve from the posterior leaf of the broad and uterosacral ligament prior to transecting the uterosacral ligament
2. Removal of the cranial part of the paracervix (including the deep uterine vein), its elevation, and dissection off the inferior hypogastric plexus
3. Transection of the uterosacral, the rectouterine, and rectovaginal ligaments between the IHP and the cervix/vagina
4. Identification and preservation of the bladder branches of the IHP before transecting the lateral leaf of the vesicouterine ligament or its transection avoiding the bladder branches of the IHP

7.4.3 Type C1 Radical Hysterectomy

The type C1 RH is a nerve-sparing operation. The superior portions of the paravaginal and pararectal spaces are fully developed to facilitate the dissection, and the ureter is completely mobilized from its bed in the paracervix and vesicouterine ligaments. The lateral resection of the paracervix involves only its cranial, "vascular" portion. As a general rule, resection of the adjacent vagina and the corresponding paracolpos is limited to 1.5–2 cm. The uterosacral ligaments are transected at the rectum, the medial leaf of the vesicouterine ligament is transected ventrally to the ureter, and the lateral leaf is transected medially to the bladder branch of the pelvic plexus.

Compared to the type B RH, type C1 has a wider margin of resection around the cervical tumor, and, compared to the type C2 operation, it preserves the hypogastric nerve component of the uterosacral ligaments and the caudal portion of the paracervix, avoiding transection of the bladder branches of the pelvic plexus in the lateral part of the vesicouterine ligament. Consequently, the postoperative function of the bladder and rectum is in the great majority of cases satisfactory. Moreover the limited resection of the vagina, though tailored to the disease burden, preserves most of the autonomic bladder nerves and seldom shortens the vagina to cause sexual dysfunction.

The operation can be performed through a low transverse or vertical midline incision, with a minimally invasive approach depending on the patient's habitus and the risk for aortic nodal disease.

7.4.3.1 Step 1: Entering the Retroperitoneum, Developing the Retroperitoneal Spaces

- After abdominal exploration, especially of the aortic and common iliac nodes for evidence of metastatic disease, the operation is begun by dividing the round ligament or entering the retroperitoneum by an incision over the psoas muscle lateral to the external iliac vessels in order to develop the pelvic wall retroperitoneal space and to expose the ureter and iliac vessels.
- Then the upper portion of the pararectal space is developed, dissecting between the ureter and hypogastric artery, posteriorly to the uterine artery. The dissection is parallel to the sacral curve. Similarly, the anterior paravesical/paravaginal space is developed by dissecting between the umbilical artery (at the lateral border of the bladder) and the distal external iliac vein.
- Next, the posterior leaf of the broad ligament is incised, and the infundibulopelvic ligaments are transected and ligated at the pelvic brim. The adnexa are mobilized and then excised.

7.4.3.2 Step 2: Pelvic Lymph Node Dissection

The pelvic lymph node dissection may be performed before or after the radical hysterectomy in the usual fashion.

7.4.3.3 Step3: Dissection of the Bladder and Ureter

- The vesicouterine fold is incised after an upward traction is applied on both sides of the bladder flap peritoneum, and the bladder flap is dissected down to the level of its attachment to the distal cervix (vesico-cervical ligament). Once the bladder flap has been mobilized, the ureter can be dissected off.
- The proper plane of dissection *is identified against the peritoneum*, and the ureter and mesoureter are easily separated from the peritoneum.
- The hypogastric nerve is identified in the mesoureter about 2 cm below the ureter, superiorly to the anterolateral rectum. Correct exposure of medial surface of the ureter, as it enters the tunnel, is obtained by its gentle lateral traction. Such a maneuver is essential to avoid injury to the ureter by stripping its adventitia and to avoid damage to the parametrial veins.
- The plane on the lateral surface of the ureter is also carefully identified and developed. The ureteral branch of the uterine artery is clipped at the ureter and divided.
- Next, the origin of the uterine artery from the medial surface of the hypogastric artery is identified, and the artery is carefully dissected from the underlying superficial uterine vein and divided at its origin. The ureter is then dissected from the lateral wall of the tunnel with the aid of gentle ventral traction.

Fig. 7.1 Unroofing of the ureter

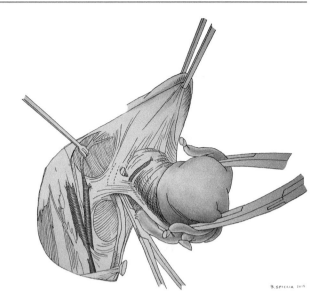

7.4.3.4 Step 4. Unroofing the Ureter

- The unroofing of the ureter is accomplished by applying Clark clamp to the tissue covering the ureter, between the ureter and the uterine artery and dividing (Fig. 7.1) the medial leaf of the vesicouterine ligament by serial clamping and cutting.
- After the ureter has been unroofed, it is retracted laterally to allow sharp dissection of the filmy attachments between the ureter and the tunnel bed to complete mobilization. Dissection of the lateral attachments of the distal ureter is not performed since it is unnecessary and will increase the risk of ureteral vascular injury.

7.4.3.5 Step 5. Division of the Cranial Part of the Paracervix

- The division of the cranial (vascular) part of the paracervix is performed by transecting one vessel at a time: the superficial uterine vein, the vaginal (inferior vesical) artery, and the deep uterine vein are successively exposed by careful dissection.

Yabuki [34, 37] described the paracervix as a lamina between the cranial part of the pararectal space and the paravesical space. The cranial part of the lamina contains not only the uterine and vaginal arteries as well as the superficial and deep uterine veins but also fatty areolar tissue with lymphatics and lymph nodes. The caudal part of the lamina containing the splanchnic nerves is referred as the lateral ligament or rectal stalk.

Fig. 7.2 Preservation
of the most lateral portion
of the vesicouterine
ligament (paracolpos)

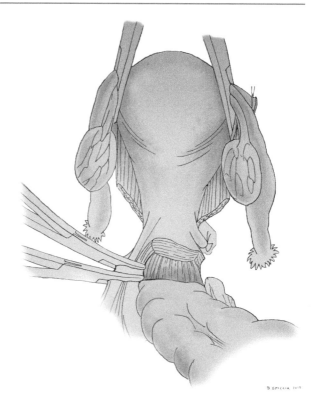

7.4.3.6 Step 6: Posterior Dissection, Division of the Uterosacral
Ligaments

- By placing traction across the posterior cul-de-sac and incising the peritoneal reflection between the rectum and the vagina, the rectal-vaginal septum is developed.
- The hypogastric nerve is dissected from the lateral aspect of the ligament before transecting the uterosacral and rectovaginal ligaments.
- The branches of the pelvic plexus to the cervix are transected with the posterior attachments of the cervix and vagina, leaving the hypogastric nerves and the pelvic plexus intact since the cranial part of the paracervix has been mobilized off the plexus.

7.4.3.7 Step 7: Dividing the Paracolpos and Vagina

- The uterus is still attached with the exception of the vagina and lateral (posterior, deep) leaf of the vesicouterine ligament (paracolpos).
- A triangular shaped view of the lateral leaf of the vesicouterine ligament bounded by the ureter, the lateral edge of the vagina and the free edge of the ligament, is better visualized when the ureter is retracted in a ventral and lateral direction and the uterus is retracted cranially.
- The most lateral portion of the ligament must be preserved since it contains the autonomic nerves to the bladder (Fig. 7.2). Whereas the medial part of the ligament adjacent to the vagina is vascular, and it can be transected, therefore preserving the

Fig. 7.3 Transection of
the medial (vascular) part
of the vesicouterine
ligament adjacent to the
vagina, preserving the
nerves to the bladder

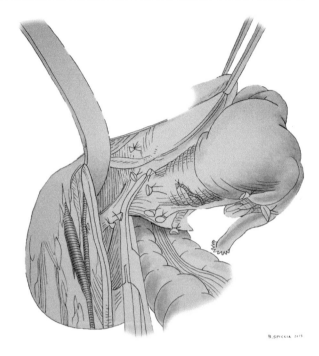

Fig. 7.4 Transection to
the vaginal wall of
remaining portions of the
rectovaginal ligament,
paracolpos, or
vesicouterine ligament still
in place

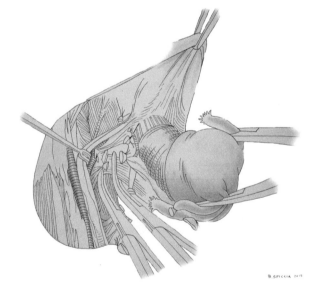

nerves to the bladder. If the remaining portions of the rectovaginal ligament, paracolpos, or vesicouterine ligament are still in place, they are transected to the vaginal
wall (Figs. 7.3 and 7.4).

7.5   Functional Outcomes

PFDs remain the major morbidity following RH. In fact, direct bladder injury and postoperative recto- and urinary-vaginal fistulas' formation are now rare. Improvements in surgical skills and technology have reduced ureteric fistula rates from 5 to 10% [13, 38] in the mid-twentieth century to less than 1% [22, 39]. However, the rate of bladder and urinary dysfunction has remained fairly constant over the last 50 years. Concerning *lower urinary tract symptoms* (*LUTS*), long-term storage, and voiding problems can be quoted around 30% after RH, even though prevalence rates from 8 to 80% are reported in the literature [22, 26, 39–41]. *Anorectal disorders* are reported within a range from 5 to 10%, being constipation the major complaint [13, 38]. Considerable *sexual dysfunctions* have also been reported after RH. A survey over 256 Swedish women with a history of early-stage cervical cancer showed reduced lubrication and moderate to much distress due to vaginal changes in one out of four of the investigated patients [15].

Obviously, any damage to the architecture of the autonomic and somatic pelvic floor innervation has a potential detrimental effect on visceral function. However, two different mechanisms prevent symptoms to occur: one is the compensatory strength intrinsic to any complex system, and the other one is neuronal plasticity as its ability to regenerate and remodeling. While thinking at pelvic floor visceral dysfunctions, one should bear in mind that symptoms occurrence is the final result of a *failed compensatory process*, not a merely result of the direct injury to a selected portion of the architecture. The concept of a *process* implies the power of neuronal plasticity and its capability to modify over time or, better, to improve the compensatory equilibrium to a point where symptoms are minimized or disappear.

The discrepancy in the prevalence data on dysfunctions (i.e., from 8 to 80% for urinary disorders) reflects the evolution and lack of consensus in surgical approach but may also enclose the different functional evaluation methods (instrumental vs clinical) and the different follow-up intervals utilized.

Comparing data from different studies is therefore extremely difficult.

Some examples of these discrepancies will help a critical understanding of the available literature.

7.5.1   Urinary Dysfunctions

A recent update on urodynamic bladder dysfunctions after RH for cervical cancer selected 19 studies from 1980 to 2010. An overall incidence of 72% of bladder dysfunctions was detected with rates for detrusor dysfunction, mixed urinary incontinence, and stress urinary incontinence of 42%, 24.5%, and 40%, respectively. Unfortunately, no data on actual symptom complaints are available; this makes difficult to understand the clinical impact of the reported figures. In addition no data on the voiding phase are mentioned in the paper [19].

On the contrary Raspagliesi et al. confine their functional assessment to bladder voiding disorders within 3 months after surgery. Comparing type II versus type III

NSRH and type III RH, they observed a prompt recovery of bladder voiding (ability to void spontaneously and post-void residual <100 ml) in type II and type III nerve-sparing surgery, differently from standard type III, where a significantly higher number of women (11/20–55 %) were discharged with self-catheterization (none and 7/59 7 %, respectively, in the other two types of RH) [23].

Again on urodynamic data, Axelsen et al. [42] compared a group of 50 women with de novo urinary incontinence versus 50 matched asymptomatic women 14 years (5–20) after RH. The only significantly different parameter between these groups was a lower maximal urethral closure pressure (MUCP) at rest and during contraction within the group of incontinent women. Additional parameters concerning the urethral pressure profile are of pathophysiological interest in this study. Unfortunately the authors missed matching the two groups for the extent of dissection during RH [42].

Conversely other authors report exclusively on symptom complaints.

A very recent prospective study adopted structured symptom questionnaires before and 6 months after laparoscopic versus abdominal RH over 54 women (27 LRH and 27 ARH). Urinary incontinence and straining during voiding were significantly more frequent after surgery in both groups (LRH, 86.9 and 34.7 %; ARH, 100 and 29.6 %). Urge incontinence, increased bladder sensation, and constipation by obstructed defecation were significantly more common postoperatively in patients undergone to ARH than after LRH [43].

Reorganization of the nervous system after trauma is a well-known phenomena [44]. Data from different studies are therefore difficult to compare because of the wide range in follow-up reported.

7.5.2   Anorectal Dysfunctions

The major complaint after RH is represented by constipation, due to a combination of slow gut transit and evacuatory difficulties (improperly termed as obstructed defecation). These problems are a spectrum ranging from patients requiring dietary changes [45] or laxatives after surgery to extreme cases in which hemicolectomies have been performed for disabling constipation [46].

Griffenberg et al. [45] reported almost 40 % of patients still experiencing bloating, abdominal discomfort, and straining at 1 year after radical surgery. Barnes et al. [13] studied anorectal physiology 1 week after surgery: rectal hyposensitivity and diminished ability of the IAS to relax to baseline were observed, although resting and squeeze pressures (functions of the IAS and EAS, respectively) were unchanged. These findings were supported by 80 % of the subjects (12/15) subjectively reporting new bowel symptoms, most commonly, loss of defecatory urge or the need to strain to defecate. However, testing anorectal physiology 6 months following radical hysterectomy over 11 women, Sood et al. [47] observed a significant decrease respect to the baseline in resting and squeeze sphincter pressures, volume of saline infused at first leak, total volume retained, and threshold volume for maximum tolerable volume (rectal hypersensitivity). The rectoanal inhibitory reflex was impaired in 64% of patients, suggesting autonomic damage. Importantly, 55% of women continued to report functional difficulties as late as 18 months, including constipation and the onset of fecal incontinence. To opposite manometric findings came Loizzi et al. [48] investigating 21 women 6 months after nerve-sparing RH: no changes from baseline were observed after surgery in any of the tested parameters, including rectal compliance.

The role of adjuvant radiation is controversial, but radiotherapy has to be considered a relevant confounding factor while investigating visceral morbidity after RH [49].

In summary anorectal neurogenic injury after RH seems to affect mainly the coordination between sensation and reflex sphincteric action, rather than simple IAS or EAS functionalities. These pathophysiological changes impact mainly on the ability to defecate with minor effect on continence and with a spectrum of symptom severity. This is a further confirmation of the concept of pelvic visceral symptoms as a *failed compensatory process*, as highlighted before.

The impact of RH on sexuality is still substantial. In a recent retrospective study comparing nerve-sparing versus standard RH (mean follow-up 31 months), overall rates of sexual dysfunctions among 114 sexually active women who responded to a questionnaire were as follows: 78% reduced sexual frequency, 55% decreased vaginal lubrication, 35% dyspareunia, and 40% pain during coitus. Authors failed finding any significant differences between the two different surgical techniques [50].

7.6   Coming to a Conclusion?

As clearly evident from the literature shortly reported above, the present knowledge on PFDs after RH is heterogeneous and very difficult to compare. Thus, the current assumption that a nerve-sparing approach reduces surgery-related dysfunctions without compromising oncologic outcomes in early-stage cervical carcinoma remains controversial.

To clarify this point, a recent meta-analysis by Kim et al. [7] compared clinical outcomes and urinary, anorectal, and sexual dysfunctions between conventional radical surgery (CRS) and nerve-sparing radical surgery (NSRS). Of course methodological aspects are the key point here: the study included a quality analysis of selected papers adopting the Newcastle-Ottawa Scale (three parameters of quality: selection, comparability, and outcome) but also checked for truly nerve-sparing technique [51]. After searching PubMed, Embase, and the Cochrane Library, 2 randomized controlled trials, 7 prospective studies, and 11 retrospective cohort studies were included with 2,253 patients from January 2000 to February 2014. Interestingly, in terms of survival, both disease-free and overall survival rates were not different between these two treatments. In terms of visceral function, the subgroup analyses demonstrated that NSRS offers a shorter duration of postoperative catheterization and reduces urinary frequency, urinary incontinence, and constipation. No differences were observed between treatments for sexual function. Crude analyses also showed decreases in blood loss, hospital stay, frequency of intraoperative complications, and length of the resected vagina in NSRS.

The authors concluded that NSRS may not affect prognosis in patients with cervical cancer, whereas it may decrease intraoperative complications and urinary and anorectal dysfunctions despite long operative time and short length of the resected vagina when compared with CRS.

Interestingly, a sparing approach mainly addressed to the parametrial extension of the resection brings to a reduction of the resected vaginal length without a significant impact on oncological outcomes. Theoretically, sparing vaginal tissue might contribute to reduce neurogenic damage from surgery, but its role in improving functional outcomes remains to be determined.

The detrimental effect of RH on sexuality seems to be unresponsive to a more respectful surgical approach to the nervous pelvic architecture. Probably the complexity here is overwhelming the power of our studies. Further investigations are very welcome on this topic.

In conclusion the detrimental impact of RH on long-term functional morbidity may be prevented with a standardized nerve-sparing surgical approach, and therefore nerve-sparing radical hysterectomy should be considered the new standard of treatment for early-stage cervical cancer.

References

1. Li H, Jia J, Xiao Y, Kang L, Cui H. Anatomical basis of female pelvic cavity for nerve sparing radical Hysterectomy. Surg Radiol Anat. 2015;37:657–65.
2. Dursun P, Leblanc E, Nogueira MC. Radical vaginal trachelectomy (Dargent's operation): a critical review of the literature. Eur J Surg Oncol. 2007;33:933–41.
3. Morice P, Castaigne D. Advances in the surgical management of invasive cervical cancer. Curr Opin Obstet Gynecol. 2005;17:5–12.
4. Parkin DM, Bray F, Ferlay J, et al. Global cancer statistics, 2002. CA Cancer J Clin. 2005;55:74–108.
5. Morrow CP. Morrow's gynecologic cancer surgery. Surgery for Cervical Neoplasia. Encinitas, CA: South Coast Medical Publishing; 2013. p. 513–698.
6. Sankaranarayanan R, Thara S, Esmy PO, et al. Cervical cancer: screening and therapeutic perspectives. Med Princ Pract. 2008;17:351–64.
7. Kim HS, Kim K, Ryoo S-B, Seo JH, Kim SY, Park JW, Kim MA, Hong KS, Jeong CW, Song YS, On behalf of FUSION Study Group. Conventional versus nerve-sparing radical surgery for cervical cancer: a meta-analysis. J Gynecol Oncol. 2015;2(26):100–10.
8. Ditto A, Martinelli F, Borreani C, Kusamura S, Hanozet F, Brunelli C, et al. Quality of life and sexual, bladder, and intestinal dysfunctions after class III nerve-sparing and class II radical hysterectomies: a questionnaire-based study. Int J Gynecol Cancer. 2009;19:953–7.
9. Kim HS, Choi CH, Lim MC, Chang SJ, Kim YB, Kim MA, et al. Safe criteria for less radical trachelectomy in patients with early-stage cervical cancer: a multicenter clinicopathologic study. Ann Surg Oncol. 2012;19:1973–9.
10. Suh DH, Kim JW, Kang S, Kim HJ, Lee KH. Major clinical research advances in gynecologic cancer in 2013. J Gynecol Oncol. 2014;25:236–48.
11. Choi SY, Lee KH, Suk HJ, Chae HD, Kang BM, Kim CH. Successful pregnancy by direct intraperitoneal insemination in an infertile patient with failure of recanalization of isthmic stenosis after laparoscopic radical trachelectomy. Obstet Gynecol Sci. 2014;57:82–5.
12. Zullo MA, Manci N, Angioli R, Muzii L, Panici PB. Vesical dysfunctions after radical hysterectomy for cervical cancer: a critical review. Crit Rev Oncol Hematol. 2003;48:287–93.

13. Barnes W, Waggoner S, Delgado G, Maher K, Potkul R, Barter J, et al. Manometric characterization of rectal dysfunction following radical hysterectomy. Gynecol Oncol. 1991;42:116–9.
14. Trimbos JB, Maas CP, Deruiter MC, Peters AA, Kenter GG. A nerve-sparing radical hysterectomy: guidelines and feasibility in Western patients. Int J Gynecol Cancer. 2001;11:180–6.
15. Bergmark K, Avall-Lundqvist E, Dickman PW, Henningsohn L, Steineck G. Vaginal changes and sexuality in women with a history of cervical cancer. N Engl J Med. 1999;340:1383–9.
16. Pieterse QD, Ter Kuile MM, Deruiter MC, Trimbos JB, Kenter GG, Maas CP. Vaginal blood flow after radical hysterectomy with and without nerve sparing. A preliminary report. Int J Gynecol Cancer. 2008;18:576–83.
17. Jackson KS, Naik R. Pelvic floor dysfunction and radical hysterectomy. Int J Gynecol Cancer. 2006;16:354–63.
18. Aoun F, van Velthoven R. Lower urinary tract dysfunction after nerve-sparing radical hysterectomy. Int Urogynecol J. 2015;26:947–57.
19. Plotti F, Angioli R, Zullo MA, Sansone M, Altavilla T, Antonelli E, Montera R, Damiani P, Benedetti Panici P. Update on urodynamic bladder dysfunctions after radical hysterectomy for cervical cancer. Crit Rev Oncol Hematol. 2011;80:323–9.
20. Burnstock G, Milner P, O'Brien B. Autonomic nervous system. In: Williams PL, Bannister LH, Berry MM, Collins P, Dyson M, Dussek JE, Ferguson MWJ, editors. Grays anatomy. New York: Churchill Livingstone; 1995. p. 1292–311.
21. Sangwan YP, Solla JA. Internal anal sphincter: advances and insights. Dis Colon Rectum. 1998;41(10):1297–311.
22. Landoni F, Maneo A, Cormio G, et al. Class II versus Class III radical hysterectomy in stage Ib–IIa cervical cancer: a prospective randomized study. Gynecol Oncol. 2001;80:3–12.
23. Raspagliesi F, Ditto A, Fontanelli R, Zanaboni F, Solima E, Spatti G, et al. Type II versus type III nerve-sparing radical hysterectomy: comparison of lower urinary tract dysfunctions. Gynecol Oncol. 2006;102:256–62.
24. Hockel M, Horn LC, Fritsch H. Association between the mesenchymal compartment of utero-vaginal organogenesis and local tumour spread in stage Ib–IIb cervical carcinoma: a prospective study [J]. Lancet Oncol. 2005;6:751–6.
25. Raspagliesi F, Ditto A, Hanozet F, et al. Nerve-sparing radical hysterectomy in cervical cancer: evolution of concepts. Gynecol Oncol. 2007;107:119–21.
26. Piver MS, Rutledge F, Smith JP. Five classes of extended hysterectomy for women with cervical cancer. Obstet Gynecol. 1974;44(2):265–72.
27. Querleu D, Morrow CP. Classification of radical hysterectomy. Lancet Oncol. 2008;9(3):297–303.
28. Fujii S. Anatomic identification of nerve-sparing radical hysterectomy: a step-by-step procedure. Gynecol Oncol. 2008;111(2 Suppl):S33–41.
29. Kato K, Suzuka K, Osaki T, Tanaka N. Unilateral or bilateral nerve-sparing radical hysterectomy: a surgical technique to preserve the pelvic autonomic nerves while increasing radicality. Int J Gynecol Cancer. 2007;17(5):1172–8.
30. Maas CP, Kenter GG, Trimbos JB, Deruiter MC. Anatomical basis for nerve-sparing radical hysterectomy: immunohistochemical study of the pelvic autonomic nerves. Acta Obstet Gynecol Scand. 2005;84(9):868–74.
31. Possover M, Quakernack J, Chiantera V. The LANN technique to reduce postoperative functional morbidity in laparoscopic radical pelvic surgery. J Am Coll Surg. 2005;201:913–7.
32. Höckel M, Horn L-C, Hentschel B, Höckel S, Naumann G. Total mesometrial resection: high resolution nerve-sparing radical hysterectomy based on developmentally defined surgical anatomy. Int J Gynecol Cancer. 2003;13:791–803.
33. Kato T, Murakami G, Yabuki Y. A new perspective on nerve-sparing radical hysterectomy: nerve topography and over-preservation of the cardinal ligament. Jpn J Clin Oncol. 2003;33:589–91.
34. Yabuki Y, Asamoto A, Hoshiba T, Nishimoto H, Nishikawa Y, Nakajima T. Radical hysterectomy: an anatomic evaluation of parametrial dissection. Gynecol Oncol. 2000;77:155–63.
35. Ercoli A, Delmas V, Gadonneix P, Fanfani F, Villet R, Paparella P, Mancuso S, Scambia G. Classical and nerve-sparing radical hysterectomy: an evaluation of the risk of injury to the autonomous pelvic nerves. Surg Radiol Anat. 2003;25:200–6.

36. Sakuragi N, Todo Y, Kudo M, Yamamoto R, Sato T. A systematic nerve-sparing radical hysterectomy technique in invasive cervical cancer for preserving postsurgical bladder function. Int J Gynecol Cancer. 2005;15:389–97.
37. Yabuki Y, Asamoto A, Hoshiba T, Nishimoto H, Kitamura S. Dissection of the cardinal ligament in radical hysterectomy for cervical cancer with emphasis on the lateral ligament. Am J Obstet Gynecol. 1991;164:7–14.
38. Samlal RAK, van der Velden J, Ketting BW, et al. Disease-free interval and recurrence pattern after the Okabayashi variant of Wertheim's radical hysterectomy for stage Ib and IIa cervical carcinoma. Int J Gynecol Cancer. 1996;6:120–7.
39. Magrina JF, Goodrich M, Weaver A, Podratz KC. Modified radical hysterectomy: morbidity and mortality. Gynaecol Oncol. 1995;59:277–82.
40. Covens A, Rosen B, Gibbons A, et al. Differences in the morbidity of radical hysterectomy between gynaecological oncologists. Gynaecol Oncol. 1993;51:39–45.
41. Massi G, Savino L, Susini T. Three classes of radical vaginal hysterectomy for treatment of endometrial and cervical cancer. Am J Obstet Gynecol. 1996;175:1576–85.
42. Axelsen SM, Bek KM, Petersen LK. Urodynamic and ultrasound characteristics of incontinence after radical hysterectomy. Neurourol Urodyn. 2007;26:794–9.
43. Laterza RM, Salvatore S, Ghezzi F, Serati M, Umek W, Koelbl H. Urinary and anal dysfunction after laparoscopic versus laparotomic radical hysterectomy. Eur J Obst Gyn Clin Reprod Biol. 2015;194:11–6.
44. De Groat WC, Kawatani M. Reorganization of sympathetic preganglionic connections in cat bladder ganglia following parasympathetic denervation. J Physiol. 1989;49:431.
45. Griffenberg L, Morris M, Atkinson N, Levenback C. The effect of dietary fibre on bowel function following radical hysterectomy: a randomized trial. Gynaecol Oncol. 1997;66:417–24.
46. Vierhout ME, Schreuder HWB, Veen HF. Severe slow transit constipation following radical hysterectomy. Gynaecol Oncol. 1993;51:401–3.
47. Sood A, Nygaard I, Shahin MS, Sorosky JI, Lutgendorf SK, Rao SSC. Anorectal dysfunction after surgical treatment for cervical cancer. Am Coll Surg. 2002;4:513–9.
48. Loizzi V, Cormio G, Lobascio PL, Marino F, De Fazio M, Falagario M, Leone L, Difiore G, Scardigno D, Selvaggi L, Altomare DF. Bowel dysfunction following nerve-sparing radical hysterectomy for cervical cancer: a prospective study. Oncology. 2014;86:239–43.
49. Yeoh E, Sun WM, Russo A, Ibanez L, Horowitz M. A retrospective study of the effects of pelvic irradiation for gynaecological cancer on anorectal function. Int J Radiat Oncol Biol Phys. 1996;35:1003–10.
50. Wang W, Li B, Zuo J, Zhang G, Yang Y, Zeng H, et al. Evaluation of pelvic visceral functions after modified nerve-sparing radical hysterectomy. Chin Med J (Engl). 2014;127:696–701.
51. Wells GA, Shea B, O'connell D, Peterson J, Welch V, Losos M, et al. The Newcastle-Ottawa Scale (NOS) for assessing the quality of nonrandomised studies in meta-analyses [Internet]. Ottawa: Ottawa Hospital Research Institute; 2014. [cited 2015 Mar 17]. Available from: http://www.ohri.ca/programs/clinical_epidemiology/oxford.asp.

Preserving Sexual Function and Continence during Radical Rectal Surgery

8

Giuseppe Cavallaro, Davide Cavaliere, and Stefano Scabini

8.1 Introduction

Since the experience reported by Heald in the early 1980s [1, 2], radical rectal surgery has dramatically changed in its functional and oncological outcomes. The identification of the so-called mesorectum and the importance of its proper fascia as an anatomical plane to be dissected and respected during radical surgery led to the standardization of a new surgical technique, the total mesorectal excision (TME), requiring a precise and diligent dissection outside the mesorectal (visceral) fascia [3]. So, excision of an intact mesorectum will therefore provide optimal surgical treatment. Local control and survival after TME are excellent in clinical series as well in large multicentric trials.

Traditionally, rectal cancer surgery is affected by high risk of sexual and urinary dysfunction, mainly related to: patient (age, sex, and cultural and psychological factors), pathology (tumor location and stage), preoperative radiotherapy. Even so, during accurate TME with respect of surgical planes, it is possible to preserve the pelvic autonomic nerves, as it is for hypogastric plexus during dissection and division of the inferior mesenteric artery [4]. Perfect knowledge of the anatomy of the pelvis and rectum is mandatory to achieve optimal oncologic and functional results.

G. Cavallaro (✉)
Department of Medico-Surgical Sciences and Biotechnologies, Sapienza University,
Rome, Italy
e-mail: giuseppe.cavallaro@uniroma1.it

D. Cavaliere
Surgery and Advanced Oncologic Therapies Unit, Morgagni-Pierantoni Hospital,
AUSL Romagna, Forlì, Italy

S. Scabini
Oncologic Surgery Unit, IRCCS San Martino Institute, Genoa, Italy

© Springer International Publishing Switzerland 2016   101
A. Carbone et al. (eds.), *Functional Urologic Surgery in Neurogenic
and Oncologic Diseases*, Urodynamics, Neurourology and Pelvic
Floor Dysfunctions, DOI 10.1007/978-3-319-29191-8_8

8.2 Surgical Anatomy: Remarks and Considerations [5–10]

The extraperitoneal rectum is embedded in a layer of fatty tissue containing draining lymph nodes and vessels (superior and middle rectal artery and vein). This layer, named mesorectum, features its own fascia, called visceral fascia (or mesorectal fascia or fascia recti). Posterolaterally, the mesorectum lines the inner pelvic wall, while anteriorly it may be covered (differently in men and women) by the peritoneal reflection and is afterward separated from seminal vesicles and prostate (in males) or from the vagina (in females) by a fibrous tissue layer called Denonvilliers' fascia (in males) and rectovaginal fascia (in females). The mesorectum gets thinner at the level of levator ani muscles and disappears at the anorectal junction.

Laterally, the mesorectum takes connection to the parietal fascia by a condensation of connective tissue (traditionally called lateral ligament), containing rectal branches of the pelvic autonomic nerve plexus and the middle rectal vessels (Fig. 8.1).

The pelvic autonomic nerve plexus includes

- Superior hypogastric plexus: located anteriorly to the body of L5, displaced on the left anterolateral side of the aorta and on its bifurcation, and represents the upper part of the pelvic plexus, being a continuation of the preaortic sympathetic plexus, originating from the spinal roots T10–L3.
- Left and right hypogastric nerves: they originate from the superior hypogastric plexus at the promontory. They run medially to the ureter and common iliac artery, going along the sidewall of the fascia recti and end as afferent fibers for the inferior hypogastric plexus. Injuries to the superior hypogastric plexus or hypogastric nerves lead to ejaculation problems, such as delayed and retrograde ejaculation, or even to urinary urgency or incontinence.

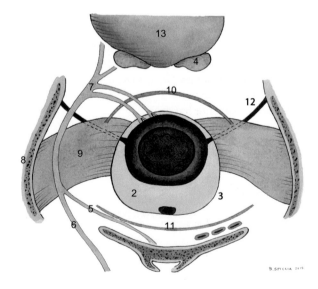

Fig. 8.1 Schematic view of mesorectum and pelvic nerves: *1* rectum, *2* mesorectum, *3* mesorectal fascia, *4* seminal vesicles, *5* erector nerve, *6* hypogastric nerve, *7* pelvic plexus, *8* pelvic wall, *9* lateral ligament, *10* Denonvilliers' fascia, *11* presacral fascia, *12* middle rectal artery, *13* bladder

- Pelvic splanchnic nerves: they originate from roots S2–S5 and contain mainly para-sympathetic fibers (erector nerves of Eckard); they are responsible for erection, detrusor contractility, vaginal lubrication, and arousal. These fibers pass through the sacral foramina, running inside the piriformis muscles and then cross the retrorectal space and form the inferior hypogastric plexus (pelvic plexus) with the hypogastric nerves. Some branches go to the rectum through the lateral ligaments.
- Inferior hypogastric plexus (pelvic plexus): formed by the joining of the hypo-gastric nerve and pelvic splanchnic nerves; it lies as a triangle in a sagittal plane at the level of S4–S5, laterally to the rectum, outside the mesorectal fascia. It ends anteriorly close to the prostate and seminal vesicles. The efferent fibers of the plexus participate to the innervation of the rectum, bladder, seminal vesicles, prostate, ureters, corpora cavernosa, uterus, and vagina. So injuries at the level of the inferior hypogastric plexus can cause erectile dysfunction, dyspareunia and impaired sensation of pain, or altered ejaculation.

Other nerves that may be involved and injured during radical rectal surgery, causing genitourinary dysfunction are

- The levator ani muscle's nerve, a motor nerve contributing to urinary continence, located within the muscle.
- The pudendal nerve, containing both somatic and sympathetic fibers originating from S1 to S5 roots. It runs into the pudendal canal to the ischioanal fossa giving branches for the pelvic floor muscles, anal sphincter, and penis or clitoris.

8.3   Technical Notes and Key Points (Fig. 8.2)

8.3.1   Ligation of the Inferior Mesenteric Artery (IMA)

IMA ligation at its origin from the aorta is a key point to obtain a complete removal of regional lymph nodes. This maneuver could lead to nerve damage, if artery dis-section is carried out without leaving a stump of at least 1–2 cm, thus preserving the preaortic and superior hypogastric plexus. Then, the presacral space at the transition between mesosigmoid and mesorectum is carefully dissected identifying and leav-ing posteriorly the hypogastric nerves.

8.3.2   Total Mesorectal Excision

During a TME, a sharp dissection is mandatory to entirely remove the rectum with respect of its visceral fascia integrity (mesorectal fascia also named fascia recti) and avoiding any infraction of the mesorectal fat tissue. These basic rules are mainstays for oncological safety when performing radical resection for rectal cancer. So the tumor and lymph nodes can be completely removed, minimizing the risk of recurrence.

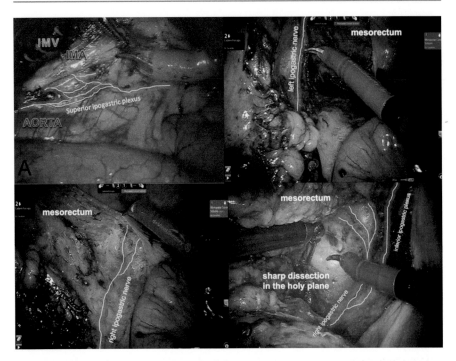

Fig. 8.2 Intraoperative views during robotic surgery: (**a**) Dissection of the inferior mesenteric artery; the superior hypogastric plexus run along the aorta; IMA should be ligated and resected at 2 cm above its own origin. (**b**) Dissection of mesorectum, left side; hypogastric nerve runs very close to the mesorectal fascia; it should be identified and lowered using a sharp dissection in the holy plane. (**c**) Dissection of mesorectum, right side: tractions and contra-tractions are essential for a correct dissection around the mesorectum. (**d**) The holy plane and pelvic nerves: the magnification and the stereoscopic view of the robotic system are useful in identification and then preservation of anatomical structures

The dissection begins posteriorly at the level of the promontory, going through the presacral space between the presacral fascia dorsally, and the mesorectal fascia ventrally, along an avascular plane, the so-called Heald's "holy plane." The superior rectal artery, situated just anteriorly to the fascia propria at the promontory, is a precise landmark for the identification of the most appropriate and safe plane of dissection. If the dissection plane lies too anteriorly, the risk is the infraction of the mesorectal fascia with higher risk of tumor spread. If the dissection lies too dorsally, there is an increased risk of bleeding and hypogastric nerves damage. These nerves run parallel to the ureter, 1–2 cm medially, underneath the internal iliac vessels, and can be followed until they get deeper into the presacral fascia (pelvic fascia) and plunge into the inferior hypogastric plexus. The posterior dissection ends at the level or rectosacral ligament. After completing this step, the dissection goes laterally dividing the so-called lateral ligaments that contain the middle rectal arteries and run close to the inferior hypogastric plexus that is rarely directly identified. At this level, care must be taken to prevent the dissection of the ligaments too close to the parietal pelvic fascia in order to avoid nerve damage.

Then the dissection goes anteriorly for the identification of the seminal vesicles and prostate, and the Denonvilliers' fascia should be always resected to obtain a proper TME. Nevertheless, many authors say that Denonvilliers' fascia resection becomes mandatory only in selected cases, given the high risk of nerve injury when entering the plane anteriorly to this fascia. For most surgeons, dissection on the mesorectal plane within its proper fascia, posteriorly to the Denonvilliers', protects the pelvic nerves and should be appropriated for posterior or posterolateral tumors; otherwise, the extramesorectal plane with resection of Denonvilliers' fascia should be considered in case of anterior or anterolateral tumors. The mesorectum ends anteriorly just below the Denonvilliers' fascia, and the correct plane of dissection lies along the muscular wall of the rectum.

8.4 Functional Results: Open and Laparoscopic Surgery

The primary aim of rectal cancer surgery is a curative resection. Even so, quality of life (QoL) may be considered as crucial as life expectancy. In particular, during surgery for rectal cancer, the maintenance of a proper genitourinary function by autonomic nerves preservation has become essential [10].

Nevertheless, even during correct TME with nerve preservation, rates of genitourinary dysfunctions remain high, particularly after abdominal-perineal resection. Before the introduction of TME technique, the incidence of postoperative voiding and sexual dysfunction was unacceptable, with reported rates from 10 to 30 % and 40–60 %, respectively. Recent studies on autonomic nerve preservation during TME have described reduced postoperative rates of voiding and sexual dysfunction in the range of 0–12 % and 10–35 %, respectively [11]. However, the real impact of the problem is probably higher, due to difficulties in conducting exhaustive clinical studies on this matter.

The COLOR II randomized trial, published in 2014 [12], compared genitourinary dysfunction after laparoscopic versus open surgery for rectal cancer. The evaluation of outcomes was made with the administration of QLQ-CR38 questionnaire before surgery and after 4 weeks, 6, 12, and 24 months. Among 617 patients enrolled (all with single rectal carcinoma located within 15 cm from the anal verge in a 2:1 ratio/randomization of laparoscopic to open), only 385 completed this phase of trial, thus confirming the difficulty to conduct functional evaluations in such patients. Genitourinary function was altered after 4 weeks in both groups (patients with a single rectal cancer within 15 cm from the anal verge), even if without significant differences. After 12 months, slight improvement in sexual function was observed. The erectile dysfunction, observed in 64.5 % of patients treated by laparoscopy and 55.6 % of patients treated by open access, worsened at 81.1 % and 80.5 %, respectively, 4 weeks after surgery and 76.3 and 75.5 % after 12 months (with no significant difference between the two groups).

A recent meta-analysis reported controversial results of laparoscopic versus open surgery. In fact, while some studies reported similar functional results (9.5 % of cases with postoperative erectile dysfunction and 3.1 % of cases with late bladder dysfunction), others report worse results in laparoscopic approach than open surgery (increase of impotence or retrograde ejaculation) [13]. Hence, it remains unclear whether a mini-invasive approach may affect genitourinary function more than open surgery, as these results may be due to limited available data or different criteria of analysis.

Urinary and sexual damage can be attributed to somatic and autonomic pelvic nerve injury during surgery. However, analyzing the functional outcomes after laparoscopic TME, we should consider that they may be biased by the multimodal therapy (preoperative chemotherapy and radiotherapy) employed in these patients and not only be directly caused only by the intraoperative preservation of the anatomy. Contin [14] compares late functional outcomes following preoperative neoadjuvant radiotherapy (RT) or combined chemoradiotherapy (CRT) plus surgery or surgery alone in the treatment of rectal cancer. This study highlighted that CRT negatively affects sexual functionality and concludes that the potential benefits of RT or CRT need to be balanced against the risk of increased genitourinary dysfunctions, independently of the surgical technique used.

Moreover, Beppu [15] compared functional outcomes after short-term versus conventional neoadjuvant therapy and TME in 104 patients, concluding that the different neoadjuvant approaches are similar in both oncologic and functional results.

Wiltink [16] analyzed data from 478 patients with a median follow-up of 14 years after neoadjuvant short-term radiotherapy plus TME versus TME alone, reporting worse outcomes (in terms of penile erection in men and dyspareunia and vaginal dryness in women) in patients submitted to neoadjuvant RT than those who underwent surgery alone. Thus, not only surgical technique and intraoperative respect of the dissection planes and autonomic nerves but also the choice and modalities of preoperative therapies play an important role in terms of functional outcomes.

Herman analyzes QoL effects of neoadjuvant CRT in locally advanced rectal cancer [17]. Global QoL showed a statistically significant and a borderline clinically significant decrease during CRT but returned to baseline 1 month after the end of treatment. As this is true for gastrointestinal symptoms, fatigue, and urinary defects, there is evidence that sexual enjoyment and sexual function remain persistently diminished after neoadjuvant CRT.

8.5 The Impact of New Technologies

8.5.1 Intraoperative Neuromonitoring

Although intraoperative identification of hypogastric plexus and nerves is possible in the majority of patients, identification of the parasympathetic and sympathetic nerves extending deeply into the pelvis appears to be more challenging [18–21]. Several studies show that electrical stimulation of such autonomic nerves produces reproducible bladder contractions that can be used to perform a nerve-sparing technique even during TME [22, 23].

The newer intraoperative neuromonitoring (IONM) systems use bipolar electric stimulation of pelvic autonomic nerves under continuous electromyography of the internal anal sphincter and manometry of the urinary bladder [20, 21].

Although functional postoperative results are encouraging, they need to be validated by prospective trials enrolling large series of patients. The available data report the safety of the IONM during rectal surgery and a significant lower rates of urinary and anorectal functional disturbances (and slight lower rates of sexual dysfunction) after surgery with IONM in comparison to "conventional" surgery [20, 21].

8.5.2 Robot-Assisted Surgery

Robot-assisted (RA) TME for rectal cancer (RC) is gaining popularity as an effective mini-invasive approach, enabling to overcome the technical limitations of conventional laparoscopy. However, it's not clear whether the undeniable technological advantage of RA surgery translates into easier preservation of neural anatomy and better saving of autonomic urogenital function.

In fact, although RA-TME generally shows better results, the differences from the standard laparoscopy are minimal and often do not achieve any concrete statistical significance.

Nonetheless, in case of obese patients, lower tumor location, and narrow pelvis dissection, the robotic approach reduces the conversion rates and the learning curve [24, 25] while maintaining unchanged short-term oncological results, but increasing the operating room time and costs.

These early results should be taken with caution as derived from the analysis of nonrandomized studies, including limited series of patients.

Currently, the only two randomized controlled trial comparing conventional laparoscopy to RA surgery for TME in RC are ongoing [26, 27], and results are not yet available; therefore we have no high level of evidence.

It is interesting to notice that although studies comparing the two main minimally invasive techniques are lacking [28–40], there are at least seven systematic reviews and meta-analysis on this subject [41–47]; however, these studies often report single-center experiences involving small groups of patients, and therefore there is a significant risk of bias and imprecision.

Focusing only on functional results, there are ten cohort studies available [10, 28, 31, 36, 38, 48–52], but only six of them compare laparoscopy to RA surgery, among which are two retrospective and four prospective evaluations. Although most of them show an overall superiority of the RA technology [42], the findings need to be confirmed by randomized controlled trials enrolling a large number of patients.

In any case, on the basis of currently available data, the incidence of urinary retention is generally lower after minimally invasive TME, both during laparoscopy and RA surgery, and often this event is not even reported with postoperative complications [31, 39, 40].

Some other studies [28, 32, 37, 48] report without significant differences between the two approaches (2.6 % in the robotic group and 2.4 % in the laparoscopic group).

Even if the analysis is restricted to the studies focused on functional aspects, three of them report better results in the RA group, with faster recovery of urinary function [49] and urological benefits both at 3, 6, and 12 months after surgery [10, 32, 49].

Fecal incontinence and constipation are only reported in one study [28], again without significant differences between the two different approaches, respectively, 2.7 % and 8.1 % after laparoscopy versus 6.8 and 13.7 % after RA resection.

Other authors analyzed the short-term results [39] and could not find such complications after minimally invasive surgery, independently from the use of RA technique.

Erectile dysfunction is reported by several authors [28, 36], but there is no mention about the method of evaluation. Conversely, only one study [49] used a structured and standardized questionnaire (IIEF) based on sexual desire; it showed a faster recovery of erectile function within 3 months from surgery in the robotic group and within 1 year in the laparoscopic group.

Moreover, the appearance of erectile dysfunction seems not to be significantly related to the extension of mesorectal resection and tumor location but rather to be ascribed to the learning curve, the excision of bulky tumor and challenging dissections [28].

Other authors [10, 32] report some benefits after RA surgery versus laparoscopy regarding sexual function at 3 and 6 months, but such differences seem to decrease over time.

Conclusions

Even if sexual, urinary, and fecal dysfunctions are sometimes important sequelae related to rectal cancer surgery, it is very difficult to have a precise idea of their occurrences. More difficult is also to compare different surgical approaches. Certainly, mini-invasive techniques magnify the imaging, and therefore well-trained surgeons may improve their results.

However, analyzing the current literature is not possible to be conclusive because

1. The population affected by rectal cancer is heterogeneous and mainly older than 65 years: to have a real pattern of genitourinary dysfunctions before surgery is not easy.
2. The QoL tests employed are often subjective: the low rate of reported complications regarding sexual dysfunction contrasted with the higher frequency of problems reported by patients in the questionnaires.
3. In the literature, we may have observed bias of methods not only in retrospective and observational studies but also in randomized clinical trials (studies which enrolled patients with high rectal cancer, laparoscopic-assisted technique, intersphincteric dissection, others).
4. Neoadjuvant therapy plays a fundamental role in genitourinary outcomes; probably, the magnified view and respect of holy plane and nervous structures are not sufficient to balance the injury of CRT, at this time indispensable in locally advanced rectal cancer.

5. A comparison between open and laparoscopic approach is very difficult and between conventional laparoscopy and robot-assisted surgery too; the expert team who have many years of experience with mini-invasive approach will never conduct a study with an "open surgery arm" to compare this aspect.

References

1. Heald RJ, Ryall RD. Recurrence and survival after total mesorectal excision for rectal cancer. Lancet. 1986;1:1479–82.
2. Heald RJ. The Holy Plane of rectal surgery. J R Soc Med. 1988;81:503–8.
3. Enker WE, Thaler HT, Cranor ML, et al. Total mesorectal excision in the operative treatment of carcinoma of the rectum. J Am Coll Surg. 1995;181:335–46.
4. Heald RJ, Moran RJ, Ryall RD, et al. Rectal cancer: the Basingstoke experience of total mesorectal excision, 1978–1997. Arch Surg. 1998;133:894–9.
5. Hraman NB. The pelvic splanchnic nerves. J Anat Physiol. 1899;33:386–99.
6. Sato K, Sato T. The vascular and neuronal composition of the lateral ligament of the rectum and the retrosacral fascia. Surg Radiol Anat. 1991;13:17–22.
7. Jones OM, Smeulders N, Wisemann O, Miller R. Lateral ligaments of the rectum: an anatomical study. Br J Surg. 1999;86:487–9.
8. Havenga K, Enker WE. Autonomic nerve preserving total mesorectal excision. Surg Clin N Am. 2002;82:1009–18.
9. Grama FA, Burcos T, Bordea A, Cristian D. Localisation and preservation of the autonomic nerves in rectal cancer surgery: technical details. Chirurgia (Bucur). 2014;109:375–82.
10. Park SY, Choi GS, Park JS, Kim HJ, Ryuk JP, Yun SH. Urinary and erectile function in men after total mesorectal excision by laparoscopic or robot-assisted methods for the treatment of rectal cancer: a case-matched comparison. World J Surg. 2014;38:1834–42.
11. Hur H, Bae SU, Kim NK, Min BS, Baik SH, Lee KY, Kim YT, Choi YD. Comparative study of voiding and male sexual function following open and laparoscopic total mesorectal excision in patients with rectal cancer. J Surg Oncol. 2013;108:572–8.
12. Andersson J, Abis G, Gellerstedt M, Angenete E, Angerås U, Cuesta MA, Jess P, Rosenberg J, Bonjer HJ, Haglind E. Patient-reported genitourinary dysfunction after laparoscopic and open rectal cancer surgery in a randomized trial (COLOR II). Br J Surg. 2014;101:1272–9.
13. Staudacher C, Vignali A. Laparoscopic surgery for rectal cancer: the state of the art. World J Gastrointest Surg. 2010;2:275–82.
14. Contin P, Kulu Y, Bruckner T, Sturm M, Welsch T, Müller-Stich BP, Huber J, Büchler MW, Ulrich A. Comparative analysis of late functional outcome following preoperative radiation therapy or chemoradiotherapy and surgery or surgery alone in rectal cancer. Int J Colorectal Dis. 2014;29:165–75.
15. Beppu N, Matsubara N, Noda M, Yamano T, Kakuno A, Doi H, Kamikonya N, Kimura F, Yamanaka N, Yanagi H, Tomita N. Short-course radiotherapy with delayed surgery versus conventional chemoradiotherapy: a comparison of the short- and long-term outcomes in patients with T3 rectal cancer. Surgery. 2015;158:225–35.
16. Wiltink LM, Chen TY, Nout RA, Kranenbarg EM, Fiocco M, Laurberg S, van de Velde CJ, Marijnen CA. Health-related quality of life 14 years after preoperative short-term radiotherapy and total mesorectal excision for rectal cancer: report of a multicenter randomised trial. Eur J Cancer. 2014;50:2390–8.
17. Herman JM, Narang AK, Griffith KA, Zalupski MM, Reese JB, Gearhart SL, Azad NS, Chan J, Olsen L, Efron JE, Lawrence TS, Ben-Josef E. The quality-of-life effects of neoadjuvant chemoradiation in locally advanced rectal cancer. Int J Radiat Oncol Biol Phys. 2013;85:e15–9.

18. Enker WE. Potency, cure, and local control in the operative treatment of rectal cancer. Arch Surg. 1992;127:1396–402.
19. Mancini R, Cosimelli M, Filippini A, et al. Nerve-sparing surgery in rectal cancer: feasibility and functional results. J Exp Clin Cancer Res. 2000;19:35–40.
20. Kneist W, Heintz A, Junginger T. Intraoperative identification and neurophysiologic parameters to verify pelvic autonomic nerve function during total mesorectal excision for rectal cancer. J Am Coll Surg. 2004;198:59–66.
21. Kneist W, Kauff DW, Juhre V, Hoffmann KP, Lang H. Is intraoperative neuromonitoring associated with better functional outcome in patients undergoing open TME? Results of a case-control study. EJSO. 2013;39:994–9.
22. Holmquist B. Electromicturition by pelvic nerve stimulation in dogs. Scand J Urol Nephrol. 1968;2:1–27.
23. Ingersoll EH, Jones LL, Hegre SS. Effect on urinary bladder of unilateral stimulation of pelvic nerves in the dog. Am J Physiol. 1957;189:167–71.
24. Akmal Y, Baek JH, McKenzie S, Garcia-Aguilar J, Pigazzi A. Robot-assisted total mesorectal excision: is there a learning curve? Surg Endosc. 2012;26:2471–6.
25. Melich G, Hong YK, Kim J, Hur H, Baik SH, Kim NK, Sender Liberman A, Min BS. Simultaneous development of laparoscopy and robotics provides acceptable perioperative outcomes and shows robotics to have a faster learning curve and to be overall faster in rectal cancer surgery: analysis of novice MIS surgeon learning curves. Surg Endosc. 2015;29:558–68.
26. Collinson FJ, Jayne DG, Pigazzi A, Tsang C, Barrie JM, Edlin R, Garbett C, Guillou P, Holloway I, Howard H, Marshall H, McCabe C, Pavitt S, Quirke P, Rivers CS, Brown JM. ROLARR: an international, multicentre, prospective, randomised, controlled, unblinded, parallel-group trial of robotic-assisted versus standard laparoscopic surgery for the curative treatment of rectal cancer. Int J Colorectal Dis. 2012;27:233–41.
27. COLRAR. A trial to assess robot-assisted surgery and laparoscopy-assisted surgery in patients with mid or low rectal cancer https://clinicaltrials.gov/show/nct01423214.
28. Patriti A, Ceccarelli G, Bartoli A, et al. Short- and medium-term outcome of robot-assisted and traditional laparoscopic rectal resection. JSLS. 2009;13:176–83.
29. Popescu I, Vasilescu C, Tomulescu V, Vasile S, Sgarbura O. The minimally invasive approach, laparoscopic and robotic, in rectal resection for cancer. A single center experience. Acta Chir Iugosl. 2010;57:29–35.
30. Baek JH, Pastor C, Pigazzi A. Robotic and laparoscopic total mesorectal excision for rectal cancer: a case-matched study. Surg Endosc. 2011;25:521–5.
31. Park JS, Choi GS, Lim KH, Jang YS, Jun SH. Robotic-assisted versus laparoscopic surgery for low rectal cancer: case-matched analysis of short-term outcomes. Ann Surg Oncol. 2010;17:3195–202.
32. Park SY, Choi GS, Park JS, Kim HJ, Ryuk JP. Short-term clinical outcome of robot-assisted intersphincteric resection for low rectal cancer: a retrospective comparison with conventional laparoscopy. Surg Endosc. 2013;27:48–55.
33. Baik SH, Kang CM, Lee WJ, Kim NK, Sohn SK, Chi HS, Cho CH. Robotic total mesorectal excision for the treatment of rectal cancer. J Robot Surg. 2007;1:99–102.
34. Bianchi PP, Ceriani C, Locatelli A, Spinoglio G, Zampino MG, Sonzogni A, Crosta C, Andreoni B. Robotic versus laparoscopic total mesorectal excision for rectal cancer: a comparative analysis of oncological safety and short-term outcomes. Surg Endosc. 2010;24:2888–94.
35. Kim YS, Kim MJ, Park SC, Sohn DK, Kim DY, Chang HJ, Nam BH, Oh JH. Robotic versus laparoscopic surgery for rectal cancer after preoperative chemoradiotherapy: case-matched study of short-term outcomes. Cancer Res Treat. 2016; Jan; 48 (1): 225-231.
36. D'Annibale A, Pernazza G, Monsellato I, Pende V, Lucandri G, Mazzocchi P, Alfano G. Total mesorectal excision: a comparison of oncological and functional outcomes between robotic and laparoscopic surgery for rectal cancer. Surg Endosc. 2013;27:1887–95.
37. Kang J, Hur H, Min BS, Lee KY, Kim NK. Robotic coloanal anastomosis with or without intersphincteric resection for low rectal cancer: starting with the perianal approach followed by robotic procedure. Ann Surg Oncol. 2012;19:154–5.

38. Erguner I, Aytac E, Boler DE, Atalar B, Baca B, Karahasanoglu T, Hamzaoglu I, Uras C. What have we gained by performing robotic rectal resection? Evaluation of 64 consecutive patients who underwent laparoscopic or robotic low anterior resection for rectal adenocarcinoma. Surg Laparosc Endosc Percutan Tech. 2013;23:316–9.
39. Kwak JM, Kim SH, Kim J, Son DN, Baek SJ, Cho JS. Robotic vs. laparoscopic resection of rectal cancer: short-term outcomes of a case-control study. Dis Colon Rectum. 2011;54: 151–6.
40. Ng KH, Lim YK, Ho KS, Ooi BS, Eu KW. Robotic-assisted surgery for low rectal dissection: from better views to better outcome. Singap Med J. 2009;50:763–7.
41. Trastulli S, Farinella E, Cirocchi R, Cavaliere D, Avenia N, Sciannameo F, Gullà N, Noya G, Boselli C. Robotic resection compared with laparoscopic rectal resection for cancer: systematic review and meta-analysis of short-term outcome. Color Dis. 2012;14:e134–56.
42. Broholm M, Pommergaard HC, Gögenür I. Possible benefits of robot-assisted rectal cancer surgery regarding urological and sexual dysfunction: a systematic review and meta-analysis. Color Dis. 2015;17:375–81.
43. Scarpinata R, Aly EH. Does robotic rectal cancer surgery offer improved early postoperative outcomes? Dis Colon Rectum. 2013;56:253–62.
44. Memon S, Heriot AG, Murphy DG, Bressel M, Lynch AC. Robotic versus laparoscopic proctectomy for rectal cancer: a meta-analysis. Ann Surg Oncol. 2012;19:2095–101.
45. Xiong B, Ma L, Huang W, Zhao Q, Cheng Y, Liu J. Robotic versus laparoscopic total mesorectal excision for rectal cancer: a meta-analysis of eight studies. J Gastrointest Surg. 2015;19:516–26.
46. Yang Y, Wang F, Zhang P, Shi C, Zou Y, Qin H, Ma Y. Robot-assisted versus conventional laparoscopic surgery for colorectal disease, focusing on rectal cancer: a meta-analysis. Ann Surg Oncol. 2012;19:3727–236.
47. Aly EH. Robotic colorectal surgery: summary of the current evidence. Int J Color Dis. 2014;29:1–8.
48. Hellan M, Anderson C, Ellenhorn JD, et al. Short-term outcomes after robotic-assisted total mesorectal excision for rectal cancer. Ann Surg Oncol. 2007;14:3168–73.
49. Kim JY, Kim NK, Lee KY, Hur H, Min BS, Kim JH. A comparative study of voiding and sexual function after total mesorectal excision with autonomic nerve preservation for rectal cancer: laparoscopic versus robotic surgery. Ann Surg Oncol. 2012;19:2485–93.
50. Luca F, Valvo M, Ghezzi TL, Zuccaro M, Cenciarelli S, Trovato C, Sonzogni A, Biffi R. Impact of robotic surgery on sexual and urinary functions after fully robotic nerve-sparing total mesorectal excision for rectal cancer. Ann Surg. 2013;257:672–8.
51. Leung AL, Chan WH, Cheung HY, et al. Initial experience on the urogenital outcomes after robotic rectal cancer surgery. Surg Pract. 2013;17:13–7.
52. Stanciulea O, Eftimie M, David L, et al. Robotic surgery for rectal cancer: a single center experience of 100 consecutive cases. Chirurgia (Bucur). 2013;108:143–51.

Psychosexual Issues and Quality of Life after Oncologic Pelvic Surgery, with Focus on Cervical Cancer

9

Alessandra Graziottin and Monika Lukasiewicz

9.1 Introduction

The extraordinary progress in oncologic surgery has blessed patients with a "second life." The minimally invasive surgery has the ambitious goal of maximizing the benefits in terms of *health expectancy*, a challenge far beyond the goal of increasing *life expectancy*.

With this perspective, women's quality of sexual life (QoL) becomes an even more urgent issue in gynecologic oncology [1–3]. The multifactorial etiology of gynecologic cancers (GC) and the increasing prevalence of such cancers at younger ages [4–6] require a comprehensive medical and psychosexual perspective. In this context, premature iatrogenic menopause is an important factor to be considered [2].

Cancers may impact *women's sexual identity, sexual function, and sexual relationships* [1, 2]. This is all the more true in gynecologic cancer (GC), as they may wound women's (and couple's) sexuality in a number of significant ways [1–3, 7–13] (Table 9.1). Unfortunately, sexual issues are still neglected during clinical consultations [9]. In Lindau et al. study [3], 74 % of patients believed their physicians should

A. Graziottin (✉)
Center of Gynecology and Medical Sexology Hospital San Raffaele Resnati, Milan, Italy

Foundation for the Cure and Care of Pain in Women – NPO, Milan, Italy
e-mail: a.graziottin@studiograziottin.it; segreteria1@studiograziottin.it;
http://www.alessandragraziottin.it; http://www.fondazionegraziottin.org

M. Lukasiewicz, MD
IInd Department of Obstetrics and Gynecology, University of Warsaw, Warsaw, Poland

Medical Center for Postgraduate Education, Belanski Hospital, Warsaw, Poland

© Springer International Publishing Switzerland 2016
A. Carbone et al. (eds.), *Functional Urologic Surgery in Neurogenic and Oncologic Diseases*, Urodynamics, Neurourology and Pelvic Floor Dysfunctions, DOI 10.1007/978-3-319-29191-8_9

Table 9.1 Main medical and sexual side effects after treatment for cervical cancers

After surgery
Radical hysterectomy
Sexual side effects
Lack of desire/interest/motivation
Decreased vaginal lubrication/dryness
Shortening of vagina
Introital and deep dyspareunia
Lack of sensations in the labia
Infertility
Urinary complications
Voiding disorders
Urinary infections
Vesical fistulae
Intestinal problems – ileus, fistulas, obstruction – wound infection
Pelvic abscesses
Ovariectomy
Iatrogenic premature ovarian failure (POF) or insufficiency (POI)
Lymphadenectomy
Leg and/or genital lymphedema, mono- or bilateral, according to the level and extension of the lymphadenectomy
After radiotherapy
Vaginal and pelvic fibrosis ("frozen pelvis")
Sexual dysfunction (vaginal dryness, narrowing/shortening of the vagina, bleeding/spotting, introital and deep dyspareunia)
Bladder and rectal complications: incontinence, cystitis, diarrhea and pain
After chemotherapy
Cosmetic issues
Iatrogenic premature menopause
Sarcopenia and fibromyalgia
Long-term peripheral neuropathies
Neuroinflammation and depression

Modified from Lukasiewicz and Graziottin [1]

discuss sex, yet such discussions did not occur in the vast majority of cases. Indeed, up to 90 % of women after GC may experience a loss in quality of life (QoL) and sexual difficulties [1–3, 7–12].

The aim of this chapter is to analyze the impact of GC on women's sexuality and discuss how to improve the psychosexual and QoL outcomes in the context of "classic" standardized treatments versus minimally invasive oncologic surgery. The paper is based on the evidence emerging from the available literature [1–132], plus the lifelong clinical experience of the authors.

9.2   Prevalence of Female Sexual Dysfunctions (FSDS) After GC

GC and its treatment can cause short- and long-term effects on sexuality, reproductive function, and overall QoL [1–3, 15–46]. In women treated for GC, available evidence indicates that:

- *Loss of sexual desire is* reported from 38.4 to 68.3% of women [1, 3, 15–46].
- *Arousal problems, with vaginal dryness and coital difficulties,* are complained of in 55–80% of women [1, 3, 15–45].
- *Orgasmic difficulties* are reported by up to 75% of patients [1, 3, 15–46].
- *Dyspareunia* in GC survivors ranges from 21.9 to 62% [1, 3, 15–46]. Comorbidity between dyspareunia and bladder symptoms can be as high as 60% [47–50].

9.3   Etiology of FSD in GC Survivors

The etiology of FSD in women with GC is multifactorial. Sexual "comorbidity," i.e., the coexistence of impairment in sexual desire/interest, arousal, and orgasm with increased dyspareunia, is significantly increased in GC survivors [1–3, 15–46].

The most relevant etiological factors are:

9.3.1   Biological

- *Cancer dependent, based on*: *cancer histotype, stage* [2], and *recurrences, if any*. Sexual outcomes improve, if minimally invasive surgery is oncologically feasible and if sexual counseling, hormone therapy, when indicated, and pelvic floor rehabilitation are *timely* provided [1, 2, 24, 27].
- *Treatment dependent*:
  - *Surgery*: sexual outcomes are different in minimally invasive oncologic surgery versus conservative versus radical, if chemotherapy (ChT) and/or radiotherapy (RT) is needed or not, if successful nerve sparing has been performed.
  Type of surgery: in general, the most radical the surgery, the higher the probability of sexual dysfunctions and bladder symptoms. The most frequent complaints include vaginal shortening, vaginal dryness (unless menopausal hormone therapy, MHT, at least topical, is *timely* prescribed), introital and deep dyspareunia, coital orgasmic difficulties, and significant bladder comorbidities [16, 19, 28, 30, 33, 35, 48–51]. Lymphedema of the lower limbs and, in a few cases, of the vulva may further significantly affect body image and body feelings, cause depression, and contribute to further reduce sexual drive/interest and motivation for sexual intimacy [52, 53]. The minimally invasive surgery may definitely sign a huge difference in terms of sexual health expectancy.

Nerve sparing: it may contribute to a better sexual function and to a more competent bladder, with reduced bladder comorbidities [54–56] (see also Chap. 6, part 1).

- *Radiotherapy*: women treated with radiotherapy alone are at a higher risk of an impaired sexual function in comparison to women not receiving radiation [57–61]:
- *Combined treatments*:
  Surgery and RT: QoL is less disrupted by surgery alone than by surgery with additional treatment modalities (ChT and/or RT) [27, 34, 57]. Minimally invasive surgery, carefully performed, provides the best sexual outcomes (see also Chap. 6, part 1).

  Radiotherapy appears to be the most insidious treatment as its impact on genital anatomy and physiology and on genital "cytoarchitecture," neurovascular function, and sexuality develops gradually. If appropriate rehabilitation is not timely started, the scarring of the irradiated tissues and the progressive shortening and stenosis of the vagina may completely prevent penetration [57–59]. Early prescription of topical and/or systemic estrogens, when indicated and oncologically appropriate, may contribute to maintaining lubrication and elasticity. Topical testosterone may further contribute to maintain a better cavernosal and vaginal vascular response [1, 2]. However, in these authors' knowledge, no controlled data are available on testosterone treatment in GC patients. Hands-on physiotherapy and vaginal molds are a critical part of the preventive strategy to minimize RT-negative outcomes.

  Surgery and ChT: the latter is usually combined with surgery in advanced GC. It leads to anemia; fatigue; hair loss and skin changes; loss of sex appeal, seductiveness, and beauty; weight changes; nausea; and diarrhea. It deeply affects body image, body feelings, and confidence on the sexual attractiveness of the woman, the partner, if any, and the "social mirror" perception [1, 2, 60, 62, 63]. Usually, ChT has the strongest impact on women's sexual identity. Peripheral neuropathies, secondary to ChT, may affect up to 40 % of cancer patients. They are underdiagnosed and undertreated, while their impact in terms of QoL can be devastating.
- *Treatment-related comorbidities* may further contribute to impair the biological basis of women's sexual function after GC diagnosis and treatment:
  Iatrogenic menopause causes intense and sudden menopausal symptoms (hot flashes, sweating, insomnia, tachycardia, joint pain, sexual dysfunctions – loss of libido, vaginal dryness, introital dyspareunia), concentration and memory difficulties, reduced assertiveness, low vital energy, loss of pubic hair, and reduced muscle mass [1, 2, 64–66], with a major impact on body image, body feelings, sexual drive, and motivation. Ovaries conservation, when oncologically feasible, should be prioritized in the surgical program.
  Infertility is a major depressing factor in childless women. Procedures for fertility preservation may modulate the QoL and sexual impact of GC treatment [32, 35, 47, 50].

Urinary incontinence is a direct consequence of the disruption of the sensory and motor nerve supply of the detrusor, with deterioration in detrusorial and urethral sphincter competence. Minimally invasive oncologic surgery (see Chap. 6, part 1) may specifically help women in protecting their urinary continence after GC.

Negative feedbacks from the genitals, secondary to anatomic changes and vulvar/genital paresthesias and/or pain, cosmetic impairment, vulvar lymphedema, vaginal dryness, anatomic vaginal changes, dyspareunia, lack of orgasm, and bladder symptoms [1, 47–51, 62–66, 71], may further worsen sexuality. They modify body image and body feelings and cause depression, loss of sex drive, and motivation. Genital lymphedema is particularly devastating and difficult to be medically treated.

Neuroinflammation and depression: a growing body of evidence indicates that neuroinflammation is the leading biological contributor of depression. Neuroinflammation is just as well of a major issue in oncologic patients [72, 73]. Inflammatory cytokines, tumor necrosis factor alpha, and many other inflammatory markers increase significantly in cancer patients, with peaks following surgery, chemo- and radiotherapies. The increase of inflammatory markers reaching the brain and the parallel hyperactivation of the microglia contribute to neuroinflammation, the powerful biological basis of depression, sleep disorders, fatigue and sickness behavior, and loss of vital energy and of sexual drive typical of the cancer treatment phase [74–76].

9.3.2 Psychosexual

Psychological distress was described in 45 % of cancer survivors [76]. Psychosexual factors may be:

- *Woman-dependent*, correlated with:
  - *Age at diagnosis*: the worst outcome is reported in younger patients who have not yet fulfilled their major life goals, like falling in love, achieving the desired career, getting married or living common law, or having children [1, 2, 63–65].
  - *Premorbid personality and sexual well-being* [1].
  - *Preexistent psychological-psychiatric problems* [36, 39].
- *Cancer and treatment dependent*: psychological distress may be exacerbated by distress combined with chronic fatigue, which is the symptom most complained of by cancer patients and the least listened to by physicians [1, 2, 8, 77, 78]. The impact of surgery, ChT, or RT on the woman's body image and body feelings further contributes [62].
- *Socioeconomic and context dependent*: poverty definitely worsens the outcomes as it makes less likely the probability of an early diagnosis, having the best surgery and follow-up treatments, using cultural awareness and economic means to

pursue the best postsurgical medical, psychosexual, and rehabilitative support. Besides, one meta-analysis shows that GC survivors are 1.4 times more likely to be unemployed than healthy women [81] and less likely to return to their job than other cancer survivors [82, 84]. Neurocognitive functions are significantly affected in patients treated with ChT [84], because of the associated neurotoxicity and neuroinflammation [71–75]. Moreover, quality of support in the couple and family and from healthcare providers is critical for the psychological outcome after treatment. Being single or in troubled/conflicting relationships further increases women's psychosexual vulnerability after GC.

9.4   QoL and Psychosexual Outcomes After GC

The psychosexual impact of GC is higher in younger couples without children or with children at primary school age. The main psychological, sexual, and relational outcomes include [1, 2, 8, 9, 18, 75, 83, 92]:

- *Psychological outcome*: sick women with cancer experience fear of death, which can marginalize the need of a sexual life for a period of time. Moreover, women who feel unattractive because of treatment side effects may feel rejected by their partners. Treatments cause a change in body image and body feelings, with a worrying sense of loss of control on their own body. Anxiety and depression usually get worse over time, when recurrences and/or persistent side effects of treatment affect women's QoL and sense of hope. *Depression* has two major contributors: a) the knowledge of having a life-threatening condition and b) the increase of inflammatory cytokines, tumor necrosis factor alpha, and many other inflammatory markers. They increase significantly in cancer patients, with peaks following surgery and chemo- and radiotherapies. This increase and the parallel hyperactivation of the microglia contribute to neuroinflammation, the powerful biological basis of depression, sleep disorders, fatigue and sickness behavior, and loss of vital energy and of sexual drive typical of the cancer treatment phase [71–73]. Inflammation is clearly the common denominator of both pain and depression, initiating the activation of several pathways that can trigger the transition from sickness to depression and from acute to chronic pain, particularly stemming from peripheral neuropathies. Understanding neuroimmune mechanisms that underlie depression and pain comorbidity may yield effective pharmaceutical targets that can treat both conditions simultaneously beyond traditional antidepressants and analgesics.
- *Sexual outcome*: women with a life-threatening condition usually feel and report loss of desire and motivation for sexual activities. Moreover, physical conditions as vaginal dryness and introital and deep dyspareunia worsen this condition causing pain, orgasmic difficulties, and physical and emotional dissatisfaction.
- *Relational outcome*: having a genital cancer may have a negative impact also on the partner and on the family. Couple problems are indeed very common in these cases, especially in younger couples, for the higher relevance that the sexual relation has in everyday life. The specific fear of being contagious to the partner, in

HPV-related cancers, and the guilty feelings in regard to past personal and partner's sexual behaviors are usually shared by patients with HPV-related cancers. Women may as well experience aggressive feelings against the partner considered responsible for the HPV infection (of having "caught" it) and the subsequent cancer.

9.4.1 Sexual Relationship Considerations: What About the Partner?

The male (and female) partner may experience sexual dysfunction, induced by the partner cancer condition (Table 9.2). Key issues of sexual partner of GC survivors are:

- *Sexual*: men may experience loss of sexual desire due to the impact of the iatrogenic menopause on her sexual appeal and the changes in the aesthetic/cosmetic appearance of the female genitals. Moreover, penetration may result

Table 9.2 Key issues of sexual partner of GC survivors

Sexual
Loss of men's sexual desire due to:
1. Impact of the iatrogenic menopause on her sexual appeal
2. Changes in the aesthetic/cosmetic/visual appearance of the female genitals
3. Type, extension, and duration of treatment
4. Recurrences, for their specific negative burden on the psychosexual adjustment and potential for hope in both partners
Difficulty in penetration because of vaginal dryness, stenosis, retraction, and the feeling of vaginal shortness
Loss of pleasure in oral sex because of:
Loss of the "scent of woman" due to changes in genital scent caused by premature menopause, loss of estrogens, and related changes in the vaginal ecosystem and perfume of vaginal secretions
Changes in the taste of vulvar skin and vaginal secretions for loss of sexual hormones and aversive taste of vaginal creams and suppositories
Her loss of interest in sex due to fatigue, iron deficiency anemia, loss of energy, depression, and pain
Her orgasmic difficulties because of loss of testosterone (after ovariectomy or ChT or RT) and consequences of treatment
Fear about his ability to obtain or sustain an erection; vaginal dryness itself can challenge the quality of the erection and can be perceived as a sign of sexual refusal
Psychosocial
Difficulties in communication about sexual difficulties for
The taboo of discussing intimate sexual issues
The fear of hurting the cancer survivor or be perceived as "unsensitive"
Reactive anxiety, depression, and uncertainty about the future
Fears and concerns related to additional roles and family responsibilities
Feelings of guilt about wanting to increase sexual intimacy or having a new partner

Modified from Lukasiewicz and Graziottin [1]

very difficult because of vaginal dryness, stenosis, retraction, and the feeling of vaginal shortness. Premature menopause, loss of estrogens, and related changes in the vaginal ecosystem may change the perfume of vaginal secretions causing a loss of pleasure in oral sex because of the loss of the "scent of woman" and of the lovely arousing taste of natural vaginal secretions.

- The woman's loss of interest in sex due to fatigue, loss of energy, depression, and orgasmic difficulties because of consequences of treatment may impact on male arousal and cause difficulty to obtain or sustain an erection. Vaginal dryness may be perceived as a sign of sexual refusal and/or an indication of the "insensitivity" of his sexual request and approach.

- *Psychosocial*: psychological intimacy may be impaired during important health issues as in the case of cancer. It is very difficult for the partner to communicate his concerns to the physician, in the presence of the partner, due to fear of hurting the cancer survivor. The possibility and usefulness of individual consultations for the partner should always be considered and offered. The inability in communicating may lead to reactive anxiety and depression. Moreover, uncertainty about the future leads to fears and concerns related to additional roles and family responsibilities during diagnosis, treatment, and recovery. Finally, it is not uncommon for the partner to experience feelings of guilt about wanting to increase sexual intimacy or having a new partner and to have difficulties in coping with the illness of the partner and the "burden" of the family [2]. The main worries of partners of GC survivors are usually more intense in the case of limited/absent communication [10, 23, 60, 61, 63, 76, 83, 92]: 50% of younger patients felt that more information about sexual changes should have been given to their husbands as well [93], to improve sexual outcomes [17].

9.5   Sexual Rehabilitation After Cancer Treatment

The Scenario First: The Challenge of Avoiding a Minimalistic Approach
1. *Avoiding the "collusion of silence"*: The first step to treatment is avoiding the collusion of silence between the woman and her physician. The majority of women think that vaginal atrophy and vulvar pain are normal and an ineluctable event during and after GC treatments. It is the physician's responsibility to raise the problem, but it is rarely done: *50% of physicians **do not** raise the subject*, and *only 14% of women who did discuss symptoms received a diagnosis and an effective treatment* [94].

    Before surgery, sexuality issues should be explained to the patients. A well-trained psycho-oncologist or nurse can immensely help patients with an early conversation on sexual issues. This intervention can turn into a main predictor of post-diagnosis marital adjustment [1, 10, 13].
2. *Avoiding minimalistic treatment*: what happens when a sexual problem is raised? Are we able to treat it? The second step is avoiding the minimalistic treatment: the majority of women facing a GC and asking (when asking) for solutions for their sexual concerns receive a lubricant as an answer. This is perceived as

humiliating by the woman and as a deception by the man. Not only is a lubricant not enough to rehabilitate the female genital tract, as it is like lubricating a rigid tube, but it is also perceived as a humiliating *fiction of arousal* by the couple.

9.6 Treatment Strategies

During Surgery
- Sentinel node biopsy to avoid leg lymphedema is to be recommended when oncologically appropriate.
- Nerve-sparing techniques are indicated to preserve bladder function and sexuality (see Chap. 6, part 1).
- Ovary conservation, when oncologically adequate, prevents premature menopause and maintains a better sexual function and body image.

9.6.1 After Surgery: Pharmacologic Treatments

- *Hormones* (Box 9.1):
  - *Topical estrogens* (estradiol, estriol, promestriene, conjugated estrogens) should be prescribed *soon after* surgery more so if a shortened vagina after CC, in case of cervical squamous carcinoma [95–97] or vulvar/vaginal atrophy (VVA), is present. Estriol has 1/80 of estradiol potency, and it is the safest estrogen (as it has a prominent action on estrogen receptor beta, which have antiproliferative and reparative actions). It can be used in a form of vaginal gel or vaginal suppositories, every other day, to maintain vaginal and bladder trophism. Estrogens have an effect on vaginal epithelium, diminishing postmenopausal vulvovaginal atrophy (VVA), protecting the normal pH and vaginal microbiota ("healthy biofilm") [98], and thus decreasing the incidence of *E. coli* vaginitis and lower urinary tract infections (UTIs). They also have a protective effect on urethra and bladder, thus reducing urinary incontinence, overactive bladder, and recurrent postcoital cystitis that are complained of 24–72 h after the intercourse [99–102].
  - *Systemic estrogens*: after hysterectomy, women can use only estrogens (without progesterone/progestins as they are indicated only to protect the endometrium). The good news for women and clinicians is that the Women's Health Initiative (WHI) study clearly indicated that the postmenopausal treatment with only estrogens in hysterectomized women significantly *reduces* the risk of breast cancer, while it maintains all the benefits on the cardiovascular system, brain, bones, joints, gastrointestinal, urogenital system, and sensory organs, the skin and mucosae first. It can therefore be used in the long term, if symptoms persist. However, as the systemic administration may not be sufficient to guarantee a normal vaginal lubrication [103], topical estrogens should be added to optimize the functional outcome. Hormones are indicated after squamous cell carcinoma of the cervix or if bilateral ovariectomy (for cancers different from adenocarcinomas) has been performed.

– *Testosterone*: for topical use, in the form of cream of testosterone propionate (2 %) or testosterone of vegetal derivative in Pentravan, a liposomic cream that maximizes transdermal and transmucosal treatment. Testosterone is indicated not only after ovariectomy [104] but also after pelvic radiotherapy or chemotherapy, as both destroy the ovarian Leydig cells, testosterone producers. In all these cases, women lose more than 80 % of the total testosterone with sexual symptoms (loss of desire/interest and drive, loss of systemic and genital arousal, reduced lubrication and cavernosal congestion, impaired orgasm) and systemic symptoms (depression, low vital energy, fatigue) unless testosterone is replaced. After 3 months of topical treatment, women report a more rapid genital congestion, more intense feelings of pleasure, and a reassuring orgasm "comeback." Partner reports that the physical response of the woman is more gratifying for both partners. Anecdotally, many partners report that with appropriate topical testosterone treatment, even the scent and taste of vaginal secretions and vulvar skin are much more pleasurable.
– *DHEA in cream* applied in the vagina is another useful tool to be explored in treatment. Preliminary data are very positive in terms of vaginal lubrication [105].
– *DHEA systemic (10 or 25 mg)*. Evidence-based data suggest a modest systemic effect, but the majority of women in the clinical setting report more energy, more positive feelings, increased muscle tone and strength (contrasting the sarcopenia typical of aging, menopause, and hospitalization, during cancer treatment), and an overall positive impact on mood and sexuality too. With appropriate clinical skill, the clinician can tailor the hormonal treatment according to the woman's expectations with excellent results in terms of QoL and sexual well-being [106].

Box 9.1: Time Is Key

• The *window of opportunity* concept, well accepted for postmenopausal hormone use to prevent/reduce cardiovascular and brain problems, is even more true for the vaginal dryness and atrophy after oncological gynecological treatment: "the sooner the better" is the motto. The delay in the hormonal treatment, at least vaginal, leads to nonreversible atrophic changes, tissue retraction, and scarring, particularly after radiotherapy, that would affect forever the woman's sexual life.
• *Lifelong treatment is key*, as women need *vaginal estrogens*, until the end of their life. When oncologically appropriate, topical hormonal treatments (such as estriol in gel) should be considered lifelong, if the goal is to prevent and cure the vaginal/bladder consequences of menopausal estrogen loss and of oncological treatments that further threaten the woman and couple's sexual health.

- *Nonhormonal treatments*: nonhormonal drugs (antidepressant, lubricants, hypnotics, etc.) can be considered in hormone-dependent cancers to ease menopausal and sexual symptoms.

9.7   Tips and Tricks for a Better QoL and Sexual Survival After GC

Doctor, please, what can I do to feel better and reduce all these symptoms that kill me much more than my cancer?

This is the request so many women ask their listening physician after the traumatic experience of having cancer and undergone variably aggressive treatments.

Clinical experience of the authors suggests a few more – usually neglected – adds to improve women's QoL, energy, and sexuality. Controlled studies are certainly important, but a huge clinical experience may offer some distilled tips hopefully useful in the office practice. They include, but are not limited to:

- *Treat iron deficiency anemia (IDA)* [107]: IDA is frequently present in cancer patients as a consequence of inadequate iron intake, increased losses, and side effects of treatment. The relationship of iron to brain function, cognition, and behavior, including affective behavior, is increasingly recognized [108]. IDA is associated with low mood, which further impair the coping attitudes after cancer [109]. Disturbances in iron metabolism have been suggested as potential pathological markers in depressed patients [110, 111]. IDA is correlated to chronic fatigue, which may exacerbate depressive symptoms and inertia. When considering QoL and sexual rehabilitation after cancer, it is important to make the appropriate diagnosis of comorbid iron-deficient anemia and restore adequate iron levels.
- *Treat vitamin D deficiency*: in addition to its role in calcium and bone homeostasis, vitamin D potentially regulates many other cellular functions. Observational studies suggest an association between poor vitamin D status and muscle weakness; cancer risk, including risk of recurrences; and regulation of the immune system, even if results are still contradictory and more research is needed [112, 113]. Vitamin D supplementation should be considered if the woman is found deficient after cancer treatment.
- *Antidepressants*: depression not only causes great mental anguish, but it also interferes with fundamental biological processes that regulate inflammation, coagulation, metabolism, autonomic function, neuroendocrine regulation, sleep, and appetite. The use of low-dose antidepressants, such as selective serotonin reuptake inhibitors (SSRI), has a double mechanism of action: the inhibition of the serotonin reuptake and the recognized anti-inflammatory potential of these drugs which may both contribute to treat depression due to cancer and to the general inflammatory state correlated to it [114].
- *Alpha-lipoic acid* (ALA) (300 mg twice a day, in capsules) is a potent natural antioxidant. Solid evidence shows significant benefits for symptomatic diabetic

neuropathy in several prospective, placebo-controlled studies [115]. The therapeutic action of ALA is based on its antioxidant properties [116]. It can reduce pain in multiple organs and tissues. It is of special interest in case of peripheral neuropathies after chemotherapy and/or radiotherapy. 300 mg twice a day is clinically associated with a reported improvement of peripheral paresthesias after ChT. In the clinical setting, patients acknowledge its benefits in improving symptoms of ChT-induced peripheral neuropathies.

- *Palmitoylethanolamide (PEA)* has a powerful anti-inflammatory, antalgic, and antidepressant effect as it contributes to reduce the neuroinflammation associated with cancer treatment. It has a systemic, central, and peripheral action (600 mg twice a day in capsules or sublingual) [117].
- *Hyaluronic acid* has shown [1, 2] almost the same efficacy of estriol in terms of improved lubrication and vaginal trophism, with an interesting anti-inflammatory and antalgic action. It may be administered in the form of vaginal gel or suppositories, once a day until symptom relief has been obtained and then one application every other day, in the evening. It should be considered to relieve vaginal dryness when vaginal estrogens are not indicated or the woman prefers not to use hormones.
- *Colostrum vaginal gel*: its powerful reparative action on the vagina's mucosa, due to different trophic factors, is particularly useful when vaginal dryness is complained of. Its specific therapeutic role after GCs deserves prospective controlled studies.
- *Moisturizers and lubricants* can help and are safe, but many women and partner do not like the "fiction of arousal" that lubricants give.

9.7.1 After Surgery: Nonpharmacologic Therapies

- *Physiotherapeutic rehabilitation*: Physiotherapists, but also specifically trained nurses and midwives, can have a still underappreciated role in the pelvic floor rehabilitation after GC. Specific treatment care includes a preliminary pharmacologic treatment (either hormonal or nonhormonal) of vaginal dryness. Physiotherapy includes vaginal dilators, which are recommended to reduce the impact of pelvic radiotherapy on vaginal elasticity and receptiveness [118]. Dilators and topical estrogen therapy can synergize in reducing vaginal dryness and dyspareunia. Moisturizers and lubricants can ease penetration [119]. Information about sexual rehabilitation with dilators and physiotherapy should be provided by *radiation oncologist before treatment*. Specifically *trained oncology nurses*, who are naturally more prone to deal with the intimacy of the patients, should give psychological and medical support to the use of dilators. Usually, it is suggested to start dilation 4 weeks after treatment and to perform dilation two to three times a week for 1–3 min; this therapy has to be continued for 9–12 months [120]. In the authors' practice, molds or dilators can be used earlier than 1 month. Daily use for 5 min, twice a day, provides better outcomes in terms of vaginal sexual elasticity, receptiveness, and "habitability."

- *Pelvic floor rehabilitation hands-on* may further contribute to maintain elasticity through appropriate stretching, massage, electromyographic feedback, and physiotherapy [121].
- *Regular sexual activity* (if desired) has a great benefit in preventing vaginal atrophy, once the vaginal trophism has been appropriately protected. The trophic impact of the neurovascular response associated with genital arousal is likely to promote genital neuroplasticity, endothelial trophism, and vessel plasticity.

9.7.1.1 Special Clinical Issues and Pertinent Treatments

- *If lymphedema of the lower limbs* is a concrete risk after lymph node removal, clinical recommendations include [1, 2, 52, 123]:
  - Diosmin-hesperidin treatment (two cps three times a day for 20 days, then two twice a day for 2–3 months) to improve lymph drainage
  - Daily brisk walking to facilitate lymph return
  - Lymph drainage with professional massage
  - Physiotherapy with specific techniques
  - Compressive stockings

However, the evidence on the efficacy in effectively reducing lymphedema is still limited. No specific studies on the impact of lymphedema treatment on sexual outcomes have been found.

Psychosexual Help

Brief psychosexual interventions can address the informational and sexual needs of cancer patients [124, 125]. Mindfulness training incorporated in a psychoeducational program for women with arousal disorder subsequent to gynecological cancer has been effective in preliminary studies [92, 126].

Many cancer institutions have established comprehensive multidisciplinary programs, focused on both the psychosexual and physical aspects of sexuality, with increased compliance with therapy and subjective improvement in sexual symptoms [127].

Palliative care providers can also be involved as they reassure patients and their partners that even at the end of life, when intercourse may not be feasible, physical sexual intimacy and emotional closeness can be encouraged and are worthwhile in a committed relationship.

The Challenge of Improving Lifestyles After Cancer

- *Physical exercise*: Recent studies have underlined the role of regular physical activity during and after treatment in improving cancer prognosis and overall survival, although the precise mechanisms are not fully understood. The most often cited improvements are reduced systemic and neuroinflammation, reduced depression and better immune functioning, better sleep [128], the great guardian of health and sexuality, and reduced fatigue and distress [129]. Physical activity helps to redesign the patient's body map and improve it sexually. It has an impact also on the dopaminergic system, increasing dopamine secretion critical to improve both the drive for life and for physical activity. Exercise is precious to avoid sarcopenia, which is more prevalent with increasing age, after iatrogenic menopause, and with long-lasting hospitalization due to cancer treatments.

- *Weight reduction* may improve cancer outcomes. It improves body image, self-perception, vital energy, and sex drive, especially if combined with daily physical activity. It reduces the general inflammation, decreasing the risk of depression and pain.
- *The importance of the diet*: The American Cancer Society (ACS) and the American College of Sports Medicine (ACSM) have developed nutrition and physical activity guidelines for cancer survivors based on the available evidence linking diet, weight, and physical activity to cancer outcomes [130, 131]. In addition, while the American Society of Clinical Oncology advocates secondary prevention including maintenance of healthy body weight and adoption of an active lifestyle specifically for colorectal cancer survivors [132], these guidelines should be considered universally by all survivors. Key points of the ACS/ACSM recommendations include:
  - Maintain a healthy weight and attempt weight loss if overweight or obese.
  - Adopt a physically active lifestyle engaging in at least 30 min of moderate to vigorous physical activity on five or more days of the week.
  - Consume a healthy diet, with at least five servings of fruits and vegetables per day and limited ingestion of processed foods and red meats.
  - Limit alcohol to no more than one drink/day and avoid smoking: alcohol and smoke may exacerbate inflammatory condition and have a detrimental mental effect.
- *The importance of sleeping*: protect the sleeping quality, also with the help of melatonin, a natural circadian sleep hormone [132].

Conclusions

GC may affect QoL and women's sexual identity, sexual function, and a couple's relationship both biologically and psychosocially. The goal of maintaining and restoring the best possible sexual life (penetration included!), increasing the *sexual health expectancy*, should be present in the physicians and psychosexologists' mind in every step of cancer treatment. The more this principle is respected, the better the outcome.

This chapter is extensively based on the authors' clinical experience of decades of comprehensive sexual rehabilitation after GC. The evidence supporting the pharmacologic choices is huge but usually not specifically evaluated in cancer patients. This pioneering use of many treatments in this specific field deserves clinical trials to evaluate its impact and significance in GC patients.

For example, it may be worth evaluating the best intervention for vaginal dilator use, to determine which of the minimally absorbed local vaginal estrogen products (ring, tablet, or cream) best restores vaginal integrity and sexual satisfaction and the safety of intravaginal DHEA and testosterone for this particular group. The specific role of SERMs such as ospemifene and of nonpharmacologic treatments such as ALA, PEA, and hyaluronic acid should be evaluated.

Prospective clinical trials including patient-reported outcomes are also needed to identify subgroups at higher risk of long-lasting negative consequences in terms of QoL and sexuality. Future studies should then address the impact on sexual outcome of minimally invasive oncologic surgery (see also Chap. 6, part 1).

Finally, physicians should improve their skills in discussing the sexual implications of GC. As a patient stated: "It seems unbelievable to me that a surgeon would remove one's sexual organs and never talk about sex" [3]. This is essential to help women to enjoy a more fulfilling "second life" after the challenging experience of an intimate cancer.

References

1. Lukasiewicz M, Graziottin A. Women' sexuality after gynecologic cancers. In: Studd J, Seang LT, Chervenak FA, editors. Current progress in obstetrics and gynaecology, vol. 2. 2nd ed. Mumbai: Kothari Medical; 2015 (accepted, in press).
2. Graziottin A, Lukasiewicz M. Female sexual dysfunction and premature menopause. In: Lipshultz L, Pastuszek A, Perelman M, Giraldi AM, Buster J, editors. Sexual health in the couple: management of sexual dysfunction in men and women. Verlag, New York: Springer; 2015 (accepted, in press).
3. Lindau ST, Gavrilova N, Anderson D. Sexual morbidity in very long survivors of vaginal cancer: a comparison to national norms. Gynecol Oncol. 2007;106(2):413–8.
4. Ferlay J, Shin HR, Bray F, et al. Internet. Lyon: International Agency for Research on Cancer; 2010. Available from: http://globocan.iarc.fr.
5. Siegel R, Naishadham D, Jemal A. Cancer statistics, 2012. CA Cancer J Clin. 2012;62: 10–29.
6. Jemal A, Bray F, Cencer MM, et al. Global center statistics. CA Cancer J Clin. 2011;61: 69–90.
7. Carter J, Stabile C, Gunn A, et al. The psychical consequences of gynecologic cancer surgery and their impact on sexual, emotional, and quality of life issues. J Sex Med. 2013;10(1):21–34.
8. Graziottin A, Serafini A. HPV infection in women: psychosexual impact of genital wart and intraepithelial lesions. J Sex Med. 2009;6(3):633–64.
9. Maguire R, Kotronoulas G, Simpson M, et al. A systematic review of the supportive care needs of women living with and beyond cervical cancer. Gynecol Oncol. 2015;136(3):478–90.
10. Juraskova I, Butow P, Robertson R, et al. Post-treatment sexual adjustment following cervical and endometrial cancer: a qualitative insight. Psychooncology. 2003;12(3):267–79.
11. Bifulco G, De Rosa N, Tornesello ML, et al. Quality of life, lifestyle behavior and employment experience: a comparison between young and midlife survivors of gynecology early stage cancers. Gynecol Oncol. 2012;124:444–51.
12. Ekwell E, Ternestedt B, Sorbe B. Important aspects for health care for women with gynecologic cancer. Oncol Nurs Inf Forum. 2003;30:313–9.
13. Kennedy V, Abramsohn E, Makelarski J, et al. Can you ask? We just did! Assessing sexual function and concerns in patients presenting for initial gynecologic oncology consultation. Gynecol Oncol. 2015;137(1):119-24. doi: 10.1016/j.ygyno.2015.01.451. Epub 2015 Jan 9.
14. Graziottin A, Gambini D. Female sexual dysfunction: treatment. In: Bø K, Berghmans B, Mørkved S, Van Kampen M, editors. Evidence-based physical therapy for the pelvic floor – bridging science and clinical practice. 2nd ed. Oxford: Elsevier; 2015 (accepted, in press).
15. Anderson B, Woods X, Copeland L. Sexual self-schema and sexual morbidity among gynecological cancer survivors. J Consult Clin Psychol. 1997;65:221–9.
16. White ID. The assessment and management of sexual difficulties after treatment of cervical and endometrial malignancies. Clin Oncol (R Coll Radiol). 2008;20(6):488–96.

17. Tierney DK. Sexuality: a quality-of-life issue for cancer survivors. Semin Oncol Nurs. 2008;24:71–9.
18. Gilbert E, Ussher JM, Perz J. Sexuality after gynecological cancer: a review of the material, intrapsychic, and discursive aspects of treatment on women's sexual-wellbeing. Maturitas. 2011;70:42–57.
19. Lammerink E, de Bock G, Pras E, et al. Sexual functioning of cervical cancer survivors: a review with a female perspective. Maturitas. 2012;72:296–304.
20. Abbott-Anderson K, Kwekeboom KL. A systematic review of sexual concerns reported by gynecological cancer survivors. Gynecol Oncol. 2012;124:477–89.
21. Cleary V, Hegarty J, McCarthy G. Sexuality in Irish women with gynecologic cancer. Oncol Nurs Forum. 2011;38:E87–96.
22. Harter P, Schrof I, Karl LM, et al. Sexual function, sexual activity and quality of life in women with ovarian and endometrial cancer. Geburtshilfe Frauenheilkd. 2013;73:428–32.
23. Vaidakis D, Panoskaltsis T, Poulakaki N, et al. Female sexuality after female cancer treatment: a clinical issue. Eur J Gynaecol Oncol. 2014;35:635–40.
24. Bergmark K, Avall-Lundqvis E, Dickman PW, et al. Vaginal changes and sexuality in woman with a history of cervical cancer. N Engl J Med. 1999;340:1383–9.
25. Bergmark K, Avall-Lundqvist E, Dickman P, et al. Patient-rating of distressful symptoms after treatment for early cervical cancer. Acta Obstet Gynecologia Scand. 2002;443–450.
26. Jensen PT, Groenvold M, Klee MC, et al. Early-stage cervical carcinoma, radical hysterectomy, and sexual function. A longitudinal study. Cancer. 2004;100:97–106.
27. Frumovitz M, Sun CC, Schover LR, et al. Quality of life and sexual functioning in cervical cancer survivors. J Clin Oncol. 2005;23:7428–36.
28. Tangjitgamol S, Manusirivithaya S, Hanprasertpong J. Sexual dysfunction in Thai women with early-stage cervical cancer after radical hysterectomy. Int J Gynecol Cancer. 2007;17:1104–12.
29. Park SY, Bae DS, Nam JH, et al. Quality of life and sexual problems in disease-free survivors of cervical cancer compared with the general population. Cancer. 2007;110:2716–25.
30. Donovan KA, Taiaferro LA, Alvarez EM, et al. Sexual health in women treated for cervical cancer. Characteristics and correlates. Gynecol Oncol. 2007;104:428–34.
31. Burns M, Costello J, Ryan-Woolley B, et al. Assessing the impact of late treatment effects in cervical cancer: an exploratory study of women's sexuality. Eur J Cancer Care. 2007;16:364–72.
32. Pieterse QD, Kenter GG, Maas CP, et al. Self-reported sexual, bowel and bladder function in cervical cancer patients following different treatment modalities: longitudinal prospective cohort study. Int J Gynecol Cancer. 2013;23:1717–25.
33. Vistad I, Cvancarova M, Fossa SD, et al. Post radiotherapy morbidity in long-term survivors after locally advanced cervical cancer: how well do physicians' assessments agree with those of their patients? J Radiat Oncol Biol Phys. 2008;5:1334–42.
34. Greimel ER, Winter R, Kapp KS, et al. Quality of life and sexual functioning after cervical cancer treatment: a long-term follow-up study. Psychooncology. 2009;18:476–82.
35. Carter J, Sonoda Y, Baser RE, et al. A 2-year prospective study assessing the emotional, sexual, and quality of life concerns of women undergoing radical trachelectomy versus radical hysterectomy for treatment of early-stage cervical cancer. Gynecol-Oncol. 2010;119:358–65.
36. Aerts L, Enzlin P, Verhaeghe J, et al. Long-term sexual functioning in women after surgical treatment of cervical cancer stages IA to IB: a prospective controlled study. Int J Gynecol Cancer. 2014;24:1527–34.
37. Carmack Taylor CL, Basen-Engquist K, Shinn EH. Predictors of sexual functioning in ovarian cancer patients. J Clin Oncol. 2004;22:881–9.
38. Liavaag A, Dorum A, Bjoro T, et al. A controlled study of sexual activity and functioning in epithelial ovarian cancer survivors: a therapeutic approach. Gynecol Oncol. 2008;108:348–54.
39. Gershenson DM, Miller AM, Champion VL, et al. Reproductive and sexual function after platinum-based chemotherapy in long-term ovarian germ cell tumor survivors: a Gynecologic Oncology Group Study. J Clin Oncol. 2007;25:2792–7.

40. Likes WM, Stegbauer C, Tillmanns T, et al. Pilot study of sexual function and quality of life after excision for vulvar intraepithelial neoplasia. J Reprod Med. 2007;52:23–7.
41. Kim SI, Lee Y, Lim MC, et al. Quality of life and sexuality comparison between sexually active ovarian cancer survivors and healthy women. J Gynecol Oncol. 2015;26(2):148–54.
42. Aerts L, Enzlin P, Verhaeghe J, et al. Psychologic, relational, and sexual functioning in women after surgical treatment of vulvar malignancy: a prospective controlled study. Int J Gynecol Cancer. 2014;24:372–80.
43. Onujiogu N, Johvson T, Seo S, et al. Survivals of endometrial cancer: who is at risk of sexual dysfunction? Gynecol Oncol. 2011;123:356–9.
44. Aerts L, Enzlin P, Verhaeghe J, et al. Sexual functioning in women after surgical treatment for endometrial cancer: a prospective controlled study. J Sex Med. 2015;12:198–209.
45. Rowlands IJ, Lee C, Beesley VL, Australian National Endometrial Cancer Study Group, et al. Predictors of sexual well-being after endometrial cancer: results of a national self-report survey. Support Care Cancer. 2014;22:2715–2.
46. Ye S, Yang J, Cao D, et al. Quality of life and sexual function of patients following radical hysterectomy and vaginal extension. J Sex Med. 2014;11:1334–42.
47. Pieterse QD, Maas CP, Ter Kuile MM, et al. An observational longitudinal study to evaluate micturition, defecation, and sexual function after radical hysterectomy with pelvic lymphadenectomy for early-stage cervical cancer. Int J Gynecol Cancer. 2006;16:1119–29.
48. Likic IS, Kadija S, Ladjevic NG, Stefanovic A, et al. Analysis of urologic complications after radical hysterectomy. Am J Obstet Gynecol. 2008;199:644.
49. Ditto A, Martinelli F, Borreani C, et al. Quality of life and sexual, bladder, and intestinal dysfunctions after class III nerve-sparing and class II radical hysterectomies. A questionnaire-based study. Int J Gynecol Cancer. 2009;19:953–7.
50. Reid GC, DeLancey JO, Hopkins MP, et al. Urinary incontinence following radical vulvectomy. Obstet Gynecol. 1990;75:852–8.
51. Ryan M, Stainton MC, Jaconelli C, et al. The experience of lower limb lymphedema for women after treatment for gynecologic cancer. Oncol Nurs Forum. 2003;30:417–23.
52. Tiwari A, Myint F, Hamilton G. Management of lower limb lymphoedema in the United Kingdom. Eur J Vasc Endovasc Surg. 2006;31:311–5.
53. Pieterse QD, Ter Kuile MM, Deruiter MC, Maas CP, et al. Vaginal blood flow after radical hysterectomy with and without nerve sparing. A preliminary report. Int J Gynecol Cancer. 2008;18:576–83.
54. Laterza RM, Sievert KD, de Ridder D, et al. Bladder function after radical hysterectomy for cervical cancer. Neurourol Urodyn. 2015;34:309–15.
55. Bogani G, Serati M, Nappi R, et al. Nerve-sparing approach reduces sexual dysfunction in patients undergoing laparoscopic radical hysterectomy. J Sex Med. 2014;11:3012–20.
56. Katz A, Njuguna E, Rakowsky E, et al. Early development of vaginal shortening during radiation therapy for endometrial or cervical cancer. Int J Gynecol Cancer. 2001;11:234–5.
57. Nout RA, van de Poll-Franse LV, Lybeert ML, et al. Long-term outcome and quality of life of patients with endometrial carcinoma treated with or without pelvic radiotherapy in the postoperative radiation therapy in endometrial carcinoma 1 (PORTEC-1) trial. J Clin Oncol. 2011;29:1692–700.
58. Katz A. Interventions for sexuality after pelvic radiation therapy and gynecological cancer. Cancer J. 2009;15:45–7.
59. Kylstra WA, Leenhouts GHMW, Everaerd W, et al. Sexual outcomes following treatment for early stage gynecological cancer: a prospective multicenter study. Int J Gynecol Cancer. 1999;9:387–95.
60. Stead ML, Fallofield L, Selby P, et al. Psychosexual function and impact of gynecological cancer. Best Pract Res Clin Obstet Gynaecol. 2007;21:309–20.
61. Soothill K, Morris SM, Harman J, et al. The significant unmet needs of cancer patients: probing psychosocial concerns. Support Care Cancer. 2001;9:597–605.

62. Sekse RJ, Gjengedal E, Råheim M. Living in a changed female body after gynecological cancer. Health Care Women Int. 2013;34:14–33.
63. Schover LR. Premature ovarian failure and its consequences: vasomotor symptoms, sexuality, and fertility. J Clin Oncol. 2008;26:753–8.
64. Graziottin A. Effect of premature menopause on sexuality. Womens Health. 2007;3:455–74.
65. Graziottin A. Menopause and sexuality: key issues in premature menopause and beyond. In: Creatsas G, Mastorakos G, editors. Women's health and disease. Ann N Y Acad Sci. 2010;1205:254–61; available at: www.alessandragraziottin.it.
66. Oonk MH, van Os MA, de Bock GH, et al. A comparison of quality of life between vulvar cancer patients after sentinel lymph node procedure only and inguinofemoral lymphadenectomy. Gynecol Oncol. 2009;113:301–5.
67. Janda M, Obermair A, Cella D, et al. Vulvar cancer patients' quality of life: a qualitative assessment. Int J Gynecol Cancer. 2004;14:875–81.
68. Weijmar Schultz WC, van de Wiel HB, Bouma J, et al. Psychosexual functioning after the treatment of cancer of the vulva. A longitudinal study. Cancer. 1990;66:402–7.
69. Huang JJ, Chang NJ, Chou HH, et al. Pedicle perforator flaps for vulvar reconstruction – new generation of less invasive vulvar reconstruction with favorable results. Gynecol Oncol. 2015;137:66–72.
70. Graziottin A. The biological basis of female sexuality. Int Clin Psychopharm. 1998;13 Suppl 6:15S–22.
71. Graziottin A, Skaper SD, Fusco M. Inflammation and chronic pelvic pain: a biological trigger for depression in women? J Depression Anxiety. 2013;3:142–50.
72. Laviano A, Seelaender M, Rianda S, et al. Neuroinflammation: a contributing factor to the pathogenesis of cancer cachexia. Crit Rev Oncol. 2012;17:247–51.
73. Vichaya EG, Chiu GS, Krukowski K, et al. Mechanisms of chemotherapy-induced behavioral toxicities. Front Neurosci. 2015;9:131.
74. Graziottin A, Skaper SD, Fusco M. Mast cells in chronic inflammation, pelvic pain and depression in women. Gynecol Endocrinol. 2014;30:472–7.
75. Kruse JL, Strouse TB. Sick and tired: mood, fatigue, and inflammation in cancer. Curr Psychiatry Rep. 2015;17:555.
76. Zabora J, BrintzenhofeSzoc K, Curbow B, et al. The prevalence of psychological distress by cancer site. Psychooncology. 2001;10:19–28.
77. Cella DF, Wiklund I, Shumaker SA, et al. Integrating health-related quality of life into cross-national clinical trials. Qual Life Res. 1993;2:433–40.
78. Cull A, Cowie V, Farquharson D, et al. Early stage cervical cancer: psychosocial and sexual outcomes of treatment. Br J Cancer. 1993;68:1216–20.
79. Simonelli LE, Fowler J, Maxwell GL, et al. Physical sequelae and depressive symptoms in gynecologic cancer survivors: meaning in life as a mediator. Ann Behav Med. 2008;35:275–84.
80. Bourgeois-Law G, Lotocki R. Sexuality and gynecological cancer: a needs assessment. Can J Hum Sex Winter. 1999;8:231–40.L.
81. de Boer AG, Taskila T, Ojajärvi A, et al. Cancer survivors and unemployment: a meta-analysis and meta-regression. JAMA. 2009;301:753–62.
82. Ross L, Petersen MA, Johnsen AT, et al. Factors associated with Danish cancers' patients return to work. A rapport from the population-based study "The Cancer Patient's World". Cancer Epidemiol. 2011;36(2):222–9.
83. Massie MJ. Prevalence of depression in patients with cancer. J Natl Cancer Inst Monogr. 2004;(32):57–71. Review.
84. Correa DD, Hess LM. Cognitive function and quality of life in ovarian cancer. Gynecol Oncol. 2012;124:404–9. Review.
85. Sonda Y, Abu-Rustum NR, Gemignani ML, et al. A fertility-sparing alternative to radical hysterectomy: how many patients will be eligible? Gynecol Oncol. 2004;95:534–8.
86. Fast Stats; an interactive tool for access to SEER cancer statistics. Surveillance Research Program Cancer. National Cancer Institute. http://seer.cancer.gov/faststats.

87. Ng JS, Low JJ, Ilancheran A. Epithelial ovarian cancer. Best Pract Res Clin Obstet Gynaecol. 2012;26:337–45.
88. Ivanova A, Loo A, Tworoger S, et al. Ovarian cancer survival by tumor dominance, a surrogate for site of origin. Cancer Causes Control. 2015;26:601–8.
89. Forner DM, Dakhil R, Lampe B. Quality of life and sexual function after surgery in early stage vulvar cancer. Eur J Surg Oncol. 2015;41:40–5.
90. Gunderson CC, Nugent EK, Yunker AC, et al. Vaginal cancer: the experience from 2 large academic centers during a 15-year period. Low Genit Tract Dis. 2013;17:409–13.
91. Hawkins Y, Ussher J, Gilbert E, et al. Changes in sexuality and intimacy after the diagnosis and treatment of cancer: the experience of partners in a sexual relationship with a person with cancer. Cancer Nurs. 2009;32:271–80.
92. Brotto LA, Heiman IR, Goff B, et al. A psychoeducational intervention for sexual dysfunction in women with gynecologic cancer. Arch Sex Behav. 2008;37:317–29.
93. Thranov I, Klee M. Sexuality among gynecologic cancer patients – a cross-sectional study. Gynecol Oncol. 1994;52:14–9.
94. Graziottin A. The vagina' biological and sexual health: the unmet needs. Climacteric. 2015;18 Suppl 1:9–12.
95. Creasman WT, Henderson D, Hinshaw W, et al. Estrogen replacement therapy in the patient treated for endometrial cancer. Obstet Gynecol. 1986;67:326–30.
96. Michaelson-Cohen R, Beller U. Managing menopausal symptoms after gynecologic cancer. Curr Opin Oncol. 2009;21:407–11.
97. Al-Azzawi F, Bitzer J, Brandenburg U, FSD Education Team, et al. Therapeutic options for postmenopausal female sexual dysfunction. Climacteric. 2010;13:103–20.
98. Graziottin A, Zanello PP. Pathogenic biofilms: their role in recurrent cystitis and vaginitis (with focus on D-mannose as a new prophylactic strategy). In: Studd J, Seang LT, Chervenak FA, editors. Current progress in obstetrics and gynaecology, vol. 2. 2nd ed. Mumbai: Kothari Medical; 2015 (accepted, in press).
99. Graziottin A. Recurrent cystitis after intercourse: why the gynaecologist has a say. In: Studd J, Seang LT, Chervenak FA, editors. Current progress in obstetrics and gynaecology, vol. 2. 2nd ed. Mumbai: Suketu P. Kothari – TreeLife Media; 2014. p. 319–36.
100. Kuiper GG, Carlsson B, Grandien K, et al. Comparison of the ligand binding specificity and transcript tissue distribution of estrogen receptors α and β. Endocrinology. 1997;138:863–70.
101. Sites CK. Bioidentical hormones for menopausal therapy. Women's Health (Lond Engl). 2008;4:163–71.
102. Shanle E, Xu W. Selectively targeting estrogen receptors for cancer treatment. Adv Drug Deliv Rev. 2010;62:1265–76.
103. Sarrel PM. Effects of hormone replacement therapy on sexual psychophysiology and behavior in postmenopause. J Womens Health Gend Based Med. 2000;9 Suppl 1:S25–32.
104. Kotz K, Alexander JL, Dennerstein L. Estrogen and androgen hormone therapy and well-being in surgically postmenopausal women. J Womens Health (Larchmt). 2006;15:898–908. Review.
105. Archer DF. Dehydroepiandrosterone intra vaginal administration for the management of postmenopausal vulvovaginal atrophy. J Steroid Biochem Mol Biol. 2015;145:139–43.
106. Pluchino N, Drakopoulos P, Bianchi-Demicheli F, et al. Neurobiology of DHEA and effects on sexuality, mood and cognition. J Steroid Biochem Mol Biol. 2015;145:273–80.
107. Camaschella C. Iron-deficiency anemia. N Engl J Med. 2015;372:1832–43.
108. Wojciak RW. Effect of short-term food restriction on iron metabolism, relative well-being and depression symptoms in healthy women. Eat Weight Disord. 2014;19:321–7.
109. Chang S, Wang L, Wang Y, et al. Iron-deficiency anemia in infancy and social emotional development in preschool-aged Chinese Children. Pediatrics. 2011;127(4):e927–33.
110. Yi S, Nanri A, Poudel-Tandukar K, et al. Association between serum ferritin concentrations and depressive symptoms in Japanese municipal employees. Psychiatry Res. 2011;189:368–72.

111. Herbert B, Herbert C, Pollatos O, et al. Effect of short-term food deprivation on interoceptive awareness, feelings and autonomic cardiac activity. Biol Psychol. 2011;89:71–9.
112. Giovannucci E. The epidemiology of vitamin D and cancer incidence and mortality: a review (United States). Cancer Causes Control. 2005;16:83.
113. Feskanich D, Ma J, Fuchs CS, et al. Plasma vitamin D metabolites and risk of colorectal cancer in women. Cancer Epidemiol Biomarkers Prev. 2004;13:1502.
114. Gold PW, Machado-Vieira R, Pavlatou MG. Clinical and biochemical manifestations of depression: relation to the neurobiology of stress. Neural Plast. 2015;2015:581976.
115. Ziegler D, Ametov A, Barinov A, et al. Oral treatment with alpha-lipoic acid improves symptomatic diabetic polyneuropathy: the SYDNEY 2 trial. Diabetes Care. 2006;29:2365.
116. Gorąca A, Huk-Kolega H, Piechota A, et al. Lipoic acid – biological activity and therapeutic potential. Pharmacol Rep. 2011;63:849–58.
117. Skaper SD, Facci L, Giusti P. Mast cells, glia and neuroinflammation: partners in crime? Immunology. 2014;141:314–27.
118. Bakker RM, Vermeer WM, Creutzberg CL, et al. Qualitative accounts of patients' determinants of vaginal dilator use after pelvic radiotherapy. J Sex Med. 2015;12:764–73.
119. Carter J, Goldfrank D, Schover LR. Simple strategies for vaginal health promotion in cancer survivors. J Sex Med. 2011;8:549–59.
120. Bakker RM, ter Kuile MM, Vermeer WM, et al. Sexual rehabilitation after pelvic radiotherapy and vaginal dilator use: consensus using the Delphi method. Int J Gynecol Cancer. 2014;24:1499–506.
121. Herderschee R, Hay-Smith EC, Herbison GP, et al. Feedback or biofeedback to augment pelvic floor muscle training for urinary incontinence in women: shortened version of a Cochrane systematic review. Neurourol Urodyn. 2013;32:325–9.
122. Pelletier G, Ouellet J, Martel C, et al. DHEA for postmenopausal women: a review of the evidence. J Sex Med. 2012;9:2525–33.
123. Badger C, Preston N, Seers K, et al. Physical therapies for reducing and controlling lymphoedema of the limbs. Cochrane Database Syst Rev. 2004;18:CD003141.
124. Robinson JW. Sexuality and cancer. Breaking the silence. Aust Fam Physician. 1998;27:45–7.
125. Ganz PA, Greendale GA, Petersen L, et al. Managing menopausal symptoms in breast cancer survivors: results of a randomized controlled trial. J Nat Cancer Inst. 2000;92:1054–64.
126. Brotto J, Heiman J. Mindfulness in sex therapy: application for women with sexual difficulties following gynecological cancer. Sex Relat Ther. 2007;22:3–11.
127. Krychman M, Carter J, Amsterdam A. Psychiatric illness presenting with a sexual complaint and management by psychotropic medications: a case report. J Sex Med. 2008;5:223–6.
128. Bouillet T, Bigard X, Brami C, et al. Role of physical activity and sport in oncology: scientific commission of the National Federation Sport and Cancer CAMI. Crit Rev Oncol Hematol. 2015;94:74–86.
129. Schmitz KH, Courneya KS, Matthews C, et al. American College of Sports Medicine roundtable on exercise guidelines for cancer survivors. Med Sci Sports Exerc. 2010;42:1409.
130. Rock CL, Doyle C, Demark-Wahnefried W, et al. Nutrition and physical activity guidelines for cancer survivors. CA Cancer J Clin. 2012;62:243.
131. Meyerhardt JA, Mangu PB, Flynn PJ, et al. Follow-up care, surveillance protocol, and secondary prevention measures for survivors of colorectal cancer: American Society of Clinical Oncology clinical practice guideline endorsement. J Clin Oncol. 2013;31:4465.
132. Kireev RA, Vara E, Viña J, et al. Melatonin and oestrogen treatments were able to improve neuroinflammation and apoptotic processes in dentate gyrus of old ovariectomized female rats. Age (Dordr). 2014;36:9707.

Part II

Functional Urologic Surgery in Neurogenic Patients

Neurogenic Voiding Dysfunction: Pathophysiology and Classification

10

Antonio Luigi Pastore and Enrico Finazzi Agrò

The lower urinary tract works as a group of interrelated structures whose purpose is to bring about efficient and low-pressure bladder filling, low-pressure urine storage with perfect continence, and periodic voluntary urine expulsion. A simple way of looking at the pathophysiology of all types of neurogenic voiding dysfunction will be presented, followed by a discussion of the various systems of classification. Consistent with the author's philosophy and prior attempts to make the understanding, evaluation, and management of voiding dysfunction as logical as possible [1], a functional and practical approach will be favored.

10.1 Normal Lower Urinary Tract Function

As to store and periodically eliminate urine, the lower urinary tract is regulated by a complex neural control system located in the brain, spinal cord, and peripheral autonomic nerves that coordinates the activity of smooth and striated muscles of the bladder and urethral outlet. Neural control of micturition is organized as a complex hierarchic system in which spinal storage mechanisms are in turn regulated by circuitry in the rostral brainstem that initiates reflex voiding. Input from the forebrain triggers voluntary voiding by modulating the brainstem circuitry (Fig. 10.1).

The major component of the micturition switching circuit is a spino-bulbospinal parasympathetic reflex pathway that has essential connections in the periaqueductal

A.L. Pastore (✉)
Department of Medico-Surgical Sciences and Biotechnologies, Urology Unit,
Sapienza University of Rome, Corso della Repubblica 79, Latina, LT 04100, Italy
e-mail: antonioluigi.pastore@uniroma1.it

E. Finazzi Agrò
Department of Experimental Medicine and Surgery, Tor Vergata University,
V.le Oxford 81, Rome 00133, Italy

© Springer International Publishing Switzerland 2016
A. Carbone et al. (eds.), *Functional Urologic Surgery in Neurogenic and Oncologic Diseases*, Urodynamics, Neurourology and Pelvic Floor Dysfunctions, DOI 10.1007/978-3-319-29191-8_10

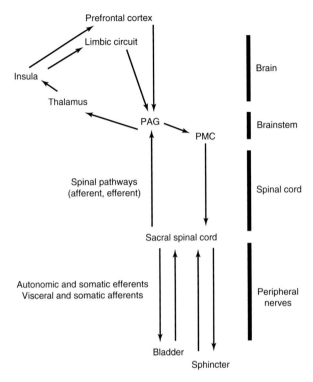

Fig. 10.1 A highly simplified model of neural control of the lower urinary tract. Afferent information is carried through visceral and somatic afferents to the spinal cord and to the periaqueductal gray and then further on to several other brain areas. The prefrontal cortex exerts tonic inhibition on the "brainstem switch" (periaqueductal gray and PMC). Receiving information on a full bladder, it decides on the social appropriateness of initiating voiding, coordinating the overall behavioral response. The limbic circuit (assessing emotional and safety homeostatic issues) may promote or inhibit "voluntary" voiding. The periaqueductal gray is the relay center for both afferent information and downstream commands. The pontine micturition center coordinates synergic voiding by simultaneously activating the bladder and the inhibiting sphincter

gray and pontine micturition center (PMC). A computer model of this circuit that mimics the switching functions of the bladder and urethra at the onset of micturition is herein described. Micturition occurs involuntarily during the early postnatal period, after which it is regulated voluntarily. Diseases or injuries of the nervous system in adults cause the reemergence of involuntary micturition, leading to urinary incontinence. The mechanisms underlying these pathologic changes are discussed.

Although disagreements exist regarding anatomic, morphologic, physiologic, pharmacologic, and mechanical details involved in both the storage and expulsion of urine by the lower urinary tract, there are points of literature agreement [1, 2]. The first is that the micturition cycle involves two relatively discrete processes: (1) bladder filling and urine storage and (2) bladder emptying. The second is that, whatever the details involved may be, one can succinctly summarize these processes from a conceptual point of view as follows:

Bladder filling and urine storage require:

1. Accommodation of increasing volumes of urine at a low intravesical pressure and with appropriate sensation
2. A bladder outlet that is closed at rest and remains so during increases in intra-abdominal pressure
3. Absence of involuntary bladder contractions

Bladder emptying requires:

1. A coordinated contraction of the bladder smooth musculature of adequate magnitude
2. A concomitant lowering of resistance at the level of the smooth and striated sphincters
3. Absence of anatomic (as opposed to functional) obstruction

The term smooth sphincter refers to a physiologic, though not anatomic, not under voluntary control (this includes the smooth musculature of the bladder neck and proximal urethra). The striated sphincter refers to the striated musculature, which is a part of the outer wall of the urethra in both the male and female (intrinsic or intramural) and the bulky skeletal muscle group that surrounds the urethra at the level of the membranous portion of the male and the middle segment in the female (extrinsic or extramural). The extramural portion, classically described as "external urethral sphincter," is under voluntary control [3, 4]. Any type of voiding dysfunction must result from an abnormality of one or more of the factors previously listed. This two-phase concept of micturition, with the three components of each related either to the bladder filling or to the outlet, provides a logical framework for a functional categorization of all types of voiding dysfunction and disorders as related primarily to filling/storage or to emptying. There are indeed some types of voiding dysfunction that represent combinations of filling/storage and emptying abnormalities. Within this scheme, however, these become readily understandable, and their detection and treatment can be logically described. All aspects of urodynamic and video urodynamic evaluation can be conceptualized exactly as what they evaluate in terms of either bladder or outlet activity during filling/storage or emptying. One can easily classify all known treatments for voiding dysfunction under the broad categories of whether they facilitate filling/storage or emptying and whether they do so by an action primarily on the bladder or on one or more of the components of the bladder outlet. Finally, the individual disorders produced by various neuromuscular dysfunctions can be thought of in terms of whether they produce primarily storage or emptying abnormalities, or a combination of the two.

10.2 Pathophysiology of Filling/Storage and Emptying Functions: Overview

Pathophysiology of the lower urinary tract may affect storage and/or voiding phase and may be secondary to reasons related to the bladder, the outlet, or both. Hyperactivity of the bladder during filling can be expressed as phasic involuntary contractions, as low compliance, or as a combination. Involuntary contractions are most commonly seen in association with neurologic disease or following neurologic injury; however, they may also be associated with aging, inflammation or irritation of the bladder wall, or bladder outlet obstruction or they may be idiopathic. Decreased compliance during filling may be secondary to neurologic disease, usually at a sacral or infrasacral level, but may also result from any process that destroys the viscoelastic or elastic properties of the bladder wall. Storage failure may also occur in the absence of hyperactivity secondary to hypersensitivity or pain during filling. Irritation and inflammation can be responsible, as well as neurologic, psychologic, or idiopathic causes. The classic clinical example is represented by interstitial cystitis.

Decreased outlet resistance may result from any process that damages the innervation, structural elements, or support of the smooth or striated sphincter. This may occur with neurologic disease or injury, surgical as well as other mechanical trauma, or aging. Assuming the bladder neck and proximal urethra as competent at rest, the lack of a stable suburethral supportive layer [5] seems a plausible explanation of the primary factor responsible for genuine stress urinary incontinence in the female. Such failure can occur because of laxity or hypermobility, both resulting in a failure of the normal transmission of intra-abdominal pressure increases to the bladder outlet. The primary etiologic factors may be any among the causes of pelvic floor relaxation or weakness. The treatment of filling/storage abnormalities is directed toward inhibiting bladder contractility, decreasing sensory input, or mechanically increasing bladder capacity or toward increasing outlet resistance, either continuously or just during increases in intra-abdominal pressure.

Absolute or relative failure to empty results from decreased bladder contractility (a decrease in magnitude or duration), increased outlet resistance, or both. Absolute or relative failure of bladder contractility may result from temporary or permanent alteration in one or more of the neuromuscular mechanisms necessary for initiating and maintaining normal detrusor contractions. Inhibition of the voiding reflex in a neurologically normal individual may also occur by a reflex mechanism secondary to painful stimuli, especially from the pelvic and perineal areas but such an inhibition may be psychogenic. Non-neurogenic causes can also include impairment of bladder smooth muscle function, which may result from over distention, severe infection, or fibrosis. Pathologically increased outlet resistance is generally seen in the male and is most often secondary to anatomic obstruction, but it may be secondary to a failure of coordination (relaxation) of the striated or smooth sphincter during bladder contraction. Striated sphincter dyssynergia is a common cause of functional (as opposed to fixed anatomic) obstruction in patients with neurologic disease or injury. The treatment of emptying failure generally consists of attempts to increase intravesical pressure or facilitate or stimulate the micturition reflex, to decrease outlet resistance, or both. If all else fail or the attempt is impractical, intermittent catheterization is an effective way of circumventing emptying failure.

Lesions of the nervous system, central or peripheral, can result in patterns of LUT dysfunction that are influenced by the level of the lesion (Fig. 10.2) [6]. Lesions of the relevant suprapontine or spinal pathways regulating LUT functions

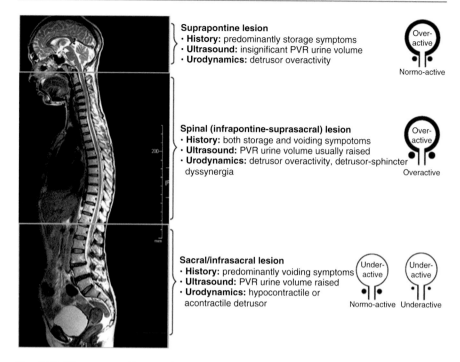

Suprapontine lesion
· **History:** predominantly storage symptoms
· **Ultrasound:** insignificant PVR urine volume
· **Urodynamics:** detrusor overactivity

Over-active

Normo-active

Spinal (infrapontine-suprasacral) lesion
· **History:** both storage and voiding sympotoms
· **Ultrasound:** PVR urine volume usually raised
· **Urodynamics:** detrusor overactivity, detrusor-sphincter dyssynergia

Over-active

Overactive

Sacral/infrasacral lesion
· **History:** predominantly voiding symptoms
· **Ultrasound:** PVR urine volume raised
· **Urodynamics:** hypocontractile or acontractile detrusor

Under-active   Under-active

Normo-active   Underactive

Fig. 10.2 The pattern of lower urinary tract dysfunction following neurologic disease is determined by the lesion site. The *blue box* represents the region above the pons, and the *green* one the sacral cord and infrasacral region. The expected dysfunctional status of the detrusor-sphincter complex is shown in figures on the right side. *PVR* post-void residual

affect the storage phase, resulting in reduced bladder capacity and detrusor overactivity, expressed as spontaneous involuntary contractions of the detrusor. The patient might report varying degrees of urinary urgency, frequency, nocturia, and incontinence (collectively known as overactive bladder symptoms). Incontinence in patients with neurologic disorders is most commonly caused by detrusor overactivity, identified by urodynamic studies. A sensation of urinary urgency is experienced as the detrusor begins to contract, and if the pressure rise continues, the patient senses impending micturition.

The mechanisms of detrusor overactivity after suprapontine damage are different from those after spinal cord injury (SCI). Damage to the suprapontine neural circuitry results in the removal of the tonic inhibition of the PMC so that spontaneous involuntary detrusor contractions occur. By contrast, the detrusor overactivity resulting from spinal cord lesions is due to the emergence of a segmental reflex at the level of the sacral cord, mediated by capsaicin-sensitive C-fiber afferents, which drive involuntary detrusor contractions. After an acute SCI, there is initially a phase of spinal shock, during which the detrusor is hypocontractile or acontractile and associated with poor bladder emptying, before spontaneous contractions occur. The duration of this phase may vary, although it is usually said to be about 6 weeks. However, during the evolution of an insidious spinal disease, the onset of detrusor overactivity can be the first observed event. The mechanism of sensitization of "silent" C fibers after SCI is uncertain; however, it is probably mediated by alterations in central synaptic connections and properties of the peripheral afferent receptors [7, 8].

Injury to the suprasacral spinal pathways also results in the loss of coordinated activation of the detrusor and inhibition of the urethral sphincter during voiding. Instead, there is a simultaneous contraction of the detrusor and urethral sphincter, known as detrusor-sphincter dyssynergia (DSD). This condition can result in voiding difficulties and incomplete bladder emptying and also dangerously high pressures in the bladder. Incomplete bladder emptying can also result from impaired parasympathetic drive caused by damage of descending bulbospinal pathways [6]. Lesions of the sacral cord or infrasacral pathways result in voiding dysfunction associated with poorly sustained or absent detrusor contractions and/or non-relaxing sphincter. Variations from these expected patterns of symptoms and findings should warrant a search for additional urological pathologies that could be occurring concomitantly.

10.3   Classification of Voiding Dysfunction

The purpose of any classification system should be to facilitate understanding and management of a dysfunction or pathology. A good classification should serve as an intellectual shorthand and should provide, in a few key words or phrases, the essence of the clinical situation. An ideal system for all types of voiding dysfunction would include or imply a number of factors:

1. The conclusions reached from urodynamic testing
2. Expected clinical symptoms
3. The approximate site and type of neurologic lesion, or lack of one

If the various categories accurately portray pathophysiology, treatment options should then be obvious, and a treatment "menu" should be evident. Most systems of classification for voiding dysfunction were formulated in order to describe dysfunctions secondary to neurologic disease or injury. The ideal system should be applicable to all types of voiding dysfunction. Based upon the data obtained from the neuro-urologic evaluation, a given voiding dysfunction can be categorized in a number of descriptive systems. In an individual patient, however, several factors define the particular state of the bladder and its outlet, and a "neurologic" classification of (neurogenic) LUTD has not been proven as clinically useful. The European Association of Urology Guidelines on Neurogenic Lower Urinary Tract Dysfunction [9] recommends the simple and therapeutically oriented Madersbacher classification system [10] for clinical practice, which differentiates between the state of the detrusor (on one side) and that of the urethral sphincter (on the other side) as either under- or overactive (or normal; Fig. 10.3). The most common dysfunction related to the nervous system lesions is an overactive detrusor with urgency, frequency,

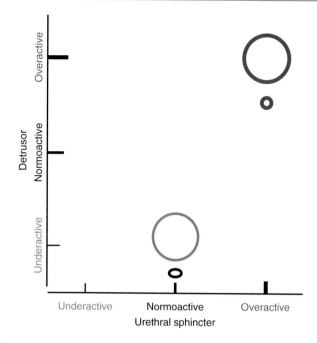

Fig. 10.3 The various patterns of neurogenic LUTD. While the normally functioning LUT is composed of a normoactive detrusor and normoactive urethral sphincter, either of these may become overactive or underactive as a consequence of neural system lesions. All different combinations of a normoactive, overactive, or underactive detrusor with a normoactive, overactive, or underactive urethral sphincter may be found in individual patients. This classification of LUTD was proposed by Madersbacher [3] and is clinically the most useful as it is directly applicable for planning rational treatment. Here, two common patterns of possible LUTD in two individual patients are shown, one demonstrating a combination of an underactive detrusor with a normoactive sphincter and the other an overactive detrusor with an overactive sphincter. The patient in the upper right corner is at risk of developing upper urinary tract involvement. The graph was constructed using the Madersbacher classification [10]

nocturia, and urge incontinence; if associated with an overactive/dyssynergic urethral sphincter, the result is high intravesical pressure leading to kidney failure.

Herein we report the most important classifications described through the years.

10.3.1 Bors-Comarr Classification

This classification system was deduced from clinical observation of patients with traumatic spinal cord injury [11]. This system applies only to patients with neurologic dysfunction and takes under consideration three principal factors:

1. The anatomic localization of the lesion
2. The neurologic completeness of the lesion
3. Whether lower urinary tract function is "balanced" or "unbalanced"

The latter terms are based solely on the percentage of residual urine relative to bladder capacity. "Unbalanced" implies greater than 20 % residual urine in a patient with an upper motor neuron (UMN) lesion or 10 % in a patient with a lower motor neuron (LMN) lesion. This relative residual urine volume was ideally meant to imply coordination (synergy) or dyssynergia of the smooth and striated sphincters during bladder contraction or attempted micturition by abdominal straining or Crede's maneuver. The determination of the completeness of the lesion is made on the basis of a thorough neurologic examination. The system erroneously assumed that the sacral spinal cord is the primary reflex center for micturition. Lower motor neuron implies collectively the preganglionic and postganglionic parasympathetic autonomic fibers that innervate both the bladder and outlet and originate as preganglionic fibers in the sacral spinal cord. The term is used in an analogy to efferent somatic nerve fibers, such as those of the pudendal nerve, which originate in the same sacral cord segment but terminate directly on pelvic floor striated musculature without the interposition of ganglia. "UMN" is used in a similar analogy to the somatic nervous system to describe those descending autonomic pathways above the sacral spinal cord (the origin of the motor efferent supply to the bladder). In this system, "upper motor neuron bladder" refers to the pattern of micturition that results from an injury to the suprasacral spinal cord after the period of spinal shock has passed, assuming that the sacral spinal cord and the sacral nerve roots are intact and that the pelvic and pudendal nerve reflexes are intact. Lower motor neuron bladder refers to the pattern resulting from damaging of the sacral spinal cord or sacral roots and when the reflex pattern through the autonomic and somatic nerves that emanate from these segments is absent. This system implies that when skeletal muscle spasticity exists below the level of the lesion, the lesion is above the sacral spinal cord and is by definition an UMN lesion. This type of lesion is characterized by detrusor hyperreflexia during filling. If flaccidity of the skeletal musculature below the level of a lesion exists, an LMN lesion is assumed to exist, implying detrusor areflexia. Exceptions occur and are classified in a "mixed lesion" group characterized either by detrusor hyperreflexia with a flaccid paralysis below the level of the lesion or by detrusor areflexia with spasticity or normal skeletal muscle tone neurologically below the lesion level.

The use of this system is illustrated as follows: a complete, unbalanced, UMN lesion implies a neurologically complete lesion above the level of the sacral spinal cord that results in skeletal muscle spasticity below the level of the injury. Detrusor hyperreflexia exists during filling, but a residual urine volume greater than 20 % of the bladder capacity is left after bladder contraction, implying obstruction in the area of the bladder outlet during the hyperreflexic detrusor contraction. This obstruction is generally due to striated sphincter dyssynergia, typically occurring in patients who are paraplegic and quadriplegic with lesions between the cervical and the sacral spinal cord. Smooth sphincter dyssynergia may also be seen in patients with spinal cord lesions above the level of T6, usually in association with autonomic hyperreflexia. An LMN lesion, complete and unbalanced, implies a neurologically complete lesion at the level of the sacral spinal cord or of the sacral roots, resulting in skeletal muscle flaccidity below that level. Detrusor areflexia results and whatever measures the patient may use to increase intravesical pressure during attempted voiding are not sufficient to decrease residual urine to less than 10 % of bladder capacity. This classification system applies best to spinal cord injury patients with complete neurologic lesions after spinal shock has passed. It is difficult to apply to patients with multicentric neurologic disease and cannot be used at all for patients with non-neurologic disease. The system fails to reconcile the clinical and urodynamic variabilities exhibited by patients who, by neurologic exam alone, seem to have similar lesions. The period of spinal shock that immediately follows severe cord injury is generally associated with bladder areflexia, whatever the status of the sacral somatic reflexes. Temporary or permanent changes in the bladder or outlet activity during filling/storage or emptying may occur secondary to a number of factors such as chronic overdistention, infection, and reinnervation or reorganization of neural pathways following injury or disease; such changes make it impossible to always accurately predict lower urinary tract activity solely on the basis of the level of the neurologic lesion. Finally, although the terms "balanced" and "unbalanced" are helpful, in that they describe the presence or absence of a certain relative percentage of residual urine, and they do not necessarily imply the true functional significance of a lesion, which depends on the potential for damage to the lower or upper urinary tracts, and also on the social and vocational disability that results.

Sensory neuron lesion		
Incomplete, balanced		
Complete, unbalanced		
Motor neuron lesion		
Balanced		
Unbalanced		
Sensory-motor neuron lesion		
Upper motor neuron lesion	Lower motor neuron lesion	Mixed lesion
Complete, balanced	Complete, balanced	Upper somatomotor neuron, lower visceromotor neuron
Complete, unbalanced	Complete, unbalanced	Lower somatomotor neuron, upper visceromotor neuron
Incomplete, balanced	Incomplete, balanced	Normal somatomotor neuron, lower visceromotor neuron
Incomplete, unbalanced	Incomplete, unbalanced	

10.3.2 The Hald-Bradley Classification

This is a simple classification exclusively based on the lesion neurotopography [12].

A supraspinal lesion implies synergy between detrusor contraction, smooth and striated sphincters, and a defective inhibition of the voiding reflex. Detrusor hyperreflexia generally occurs and sensation is usually preserved. However, depending on the site of the lesion, detrusor areflexia and defective sensation may be present. A suprasacral spinal lesion is roughly equivalent to what is described as a UMN lesion in the Bors-Comarr classification [11]. An infrasacral lesion is roughly equivalent to an LMN lesion. Peripheral autonomic neuropathy is most frequently encountered in the diabetic patients and is characterized by deficient bladder sensation, gradually increasing residual urine and ultimate decompensation, with loss of detrusor contractility. A muscular lesion can involve the detrusor itself, the smooth sphincter, or any portion, or all, of the striated sphincter. The resultant dysfunction is dependent on which structure is principally affected. Detrusor dysfunction is the most common and generally results from decompensation, following long-standing bladder outlet obstruction.

The Hald-Bradley classification
Suprasacral lesion
Suprasacral spinal lesion
Infrasacral lesion
Peripheral autonomic neuropathy
Muscular lesion

10.3.3 The Bradley Classification

This is a primarily neurologic system based upon a conceptualization of the central nervous system control of the lower urinary tract as including four neurologic "loops." Dysfunctions are classified according to the loop affected [13].

Loop 1 consists of neuronal connections between the cerebral cortex and the pontine mesencephalic micturition center; this coordinates voluntary control of the detrusor reflex. Loop 1 lesions are seen in conditions such as brain tumor, cerebrovascular accident or disease, and cerebral trophy with dementia. The final result is characteristically detrusor hyperreflexia.

Loop 2 includes the intraspinal pathway of detrusor muscle afferents to the brainstem micturition center and the motor impulses from this center to the sacral spinal cord. Loop 2 is thought to coordinate and provide for a detrusor reflex of adequate temporal duration to allow complete voiding. Partial interruption by spinal cord injury results in a detrusor reflex of low threshold and in poor emptying with residual urine. Spinal cord transection of loop 2 acutely produces detrusor areflexia and urinary retention-spinal shock. After this has passed, detrusor hyperreflexia results.

Loop 3 consists of the peripheral detrusor afferent axons and their pathway in the spinal cord; these terminate by synapsing on pudendal motor neurons that ultimately innervate periurethral striated muscle.

Loop 3 was thought to provide a neurologic substrate for coordinated reciprocal action of the bladder and striated sphincter. Loop 3 dysfunction could be responsible for detrusor-striated sphincter dyssynergia or involuntary sphincter relaxation.

Loop 4 consists of two components. Loop 4A is the suprasacral afferent and efferent innervation of the pudendal motor neurons to the periurethral striated musculature which synapse on pudendal motor neurons in Onuf nucleus – the segmental innervation of the periurethral striated muscle. In contrast to the stimulation of detrusor afferent fibers, which produce inhibitory postsynaptic potentials in pudendal motor neurons through loop 3, pudendal nerve afferents produce excitatory postsynaptic potentials in those motor neurons through loop 4B.

These provide for contraction of the periurethral striated muscle during bladder filling and urine storage. The related sensory impulses arise from muscle spindles and tendon organs in the pelvic floor musculature.

Loop 4 provides for volitional control of the striated sphincter. Abnormalities of the suprasacral portion result in abnormal responses of the pudendal motor neurons to bladder filling and emptying, manifested as detrusor-striated sphincter dyssynergia, and/or loss of the ability to voluntarily contract the striated sphincter.

This system is sophisticated and reflects the neurophysiologic expertise of its creator, Dr. William Bradley. For some neurologists, this method may be an excellent way to conceptualize the neurophysiology involved, assuming that they agree on the existence and significance of all four loops. Most urologists find this system difficult to use for many types of neurogenic voiding dysfunction and not at all applicable to non-neurogenic voiding dysfunction. Urodynamically, it may be extremely difficult to test the intactness of each loop system, and multicentric and partial lesions are difficult to describe.

10.3.4 The Lapides Classification

This is a modification of a system originally proposed by the Neurologist McLellan in 1939 [14, 15]. This remains one of the most familiar systems to urologists and non-urologists because it describes in recognizable shorthand the clinical and cystometric conditions of many types of neurogenic voiding dysfunction.

A sensory neurogenic bladder results from interruption of the sensory fibers between the bladder and spinal cord or the afferent tracts to the brain. Diabetes mellitus, tabes dorsalis, and pernicious anemia are most commonly responsible. The first clinical changes are described as those of impaired sensation of bladder distention. Unless voiding is initiated on a timed basis, varying degrees of bladder over distention can result with resultant hypotonicity. With bladder decompensation, significant amounts of residual urine are found, and, at this time, the cystometric curve generally demonstrates a large bladder capacity with a flat, high-compliance, low-pressure filling curve.

A motor paralytic bladder results from disease processes that destroy the parasympathetic motor innervation of the bladder. Extensive pelvic surgery or trauma may produce this. Herpes zoster has been listed as a cause as well, but recent evidence suggests that the voiding dysfunction seen with herpes is more related to a problem with afferent input.

The early symptoms may vary from painful urinary retention to only a relative inability to initiate and maintain normal micturition. Early cystometric filling is normal but without a voluntary bladder contraction at capacity. Chronic over distention and decompensation may occur in a large bladder capacity with a flat, low-pressure filling curve; a large residual urine may result.

The uninhibited neurogenic bladder was described originally as resulting from injury or disease to the "cortico-regulatory tract." The sacral spinal cord was presumed to be the micturition reflex center, and this "cortico-regulatory tract" was believed to exert an inhibitory influence on the sacral micturition reflex center. A destructive lesion in this tract would then result in over-facilitation or lack of inhibition of the micturition reflex. Cerebrovascular accident, brain or spinal cord tumor, Parkinson's disease, and demyelinating disease are the most common causes in this category. The voiding dysfunction is most often characterized symptomatically by frequency, urgency, and urge incontinence. Urodynamically, one sees normal sensation with an involuntary bladder contraction at low filling volumes. Residual urine is characteristically low unless anatomic outlet obstruction or true smooth or striated sphincter dyssynergia occurs. The patient generally can initiate a bladder contraction voluntarily, but is often unable to do so during cystometry because sufficient urine storage cannot occur before detrusor hyperreflexia is stimulated.

Reflex neurogenic bladder describes the postspinal shock condition that exists after complete interruption of the sensory and motor pathways between the sacral spinal cord and the brainstem. Most commonly, this occurs in traumatic spinal cord injury and transverse myelitis, but may occur with extensive demyelinating disease or any process that produces significant spinal cord destruction as well. Typically, there is no bladder sensation and there is inability to initiate voluntary micturition.

Incontinence without sensation generally occurs because of low volume involuntary bladder contraction. Striated sphincter dyssynergia is the rule. This type of lesion is essentially equivalent to a complete UMN lesion in the Bors-Comarr classification.

An autonomous neurogenic bladder results from complete motor and sensory separation of the bladder from the sacral spinal cord. This may be caused by any disease that destroys the sacral cord or causes extensive damage to the sacral roots or pelvic nerves. There is inability to voluntarily initiate micturition, no bladder reflex activity, and no specific bladder sensation. This type of bladder is equivalent to a complete LMN lesion in the Bors-Comarr classification and is also the type of dysfunction seen in patients with spinal shock. This characteristic cystometric pattern is initially similar to the late stages of the motor or sensory paralytic bladder, with a marked shift to the right of the cystometric filling curve and a large bladder capacity at low intravesical pressure. However, decreased compliance may develop, secondary either to chronic inflammatory change or to the effects of denervation/centralization with secondary neuro-morphologic and neuro-pharmacologic reorganizational changes.

Emptying capacity may vary widely, depending on the ability of the patient to increase intravesical pressure and on the resistance offered during this increase by the smooth and striated sphincters.

These classic categories in their usual settings are usually easily understood and remembered, and this is why this system provides an excellent framework for teaching some fundamentals of neurogenic voiding dysfunction to students and non-urologists. Unfortunately, many patients do not exactly "fit" into one or another category. Gradations of sensory, motor, and mixed lesions occur, and the patterns produced after different types of peripheral denervation/defunctionalization may vary widely from those which are classically described. The system is applicable only to neuropathic dysfunction.

The Lapides classification
Sensory neurogenic bladder
Motor paralytic bladder
Uninhibited neurogenic bladder
Reflex neurogenic bladder
Autonomous neurogenic bladder

10.3.5 Urodynamic Classification

Urodynamic classification systems are based solely on objective urodynamic data [16]. When exact urodynamic classification is possible, this sort of system can provide an accurate description of the voiding dysfunction that occurs. If abnormal or hyperreflexic detrusor exists with coordinated smooth and striated sphincter function and without anatomic obstruction, normal bladder emptying should occur. Detrusor hyperreflexia is mostly associated with neurologic lesions above the sacral spinal cord. Striated sphincter dyssynergia is most commonly seen after complete suprasacral spinal cord injury, following the period of spinal shock. Smooth sphincter dyssynergia is most classically in autonomic hyperreflexia when it is characteristically associated with detrusor hyperreflexia and striated sphincter dyssynergia. Detrusor areflexia may be secondary to bladder muscle decompensation or to various other conditions that produce inhibition at the level of the brainstem micturition center, the sacral spinal cord, the bladder ganglia, or the bladder smooth muscle.

This classification system is easiest to use when detrusor hyperreflexia or normoreflexia exists. Thus, a typical T-10 level paraplegic exhibits detrusor hyperreflexia, smooth sphincter synergy, and striated sphincter dyssynergia. When a voluntary or hyperreflexic contraction cannot be elicited, the application of such a system result is more difficult, since it is not appropriate to speak of true sphincter dyssynergia in the absence of an opposing bladder contraction. There are obviously many variations and extensions of such a system. Such systems work only when total urodynamic agreement exists among classifiers. Unfortunately, there are many voiding dysfunctions that do not fit completely into a urodynamic classification system that is agreed upon by all "experts." As sophisticated urodynamic technology and understanding improve, this type of classification system may supplant some others in general use.

Urodynamic classification	
Detrusor hyperreflexia (or normoreflexia)	*Detrusor areflexia*
Coordinated sphincters	Coordinated sphincters
Striated sphincter dyssynergia	Non-relaxing striated sphincter
Smooth sphincter dyssynergia	Denervated striated sphincter
Non-relaxing smooth sphincter	Non-relaxing smooth sphincter

10.3.6 International Continence Society Classification

This classification represents an extension of a urodynamic classification system. The storage and voiding phases of micturition are described separately, and, within each, various designations are applied to describe bladder and urethral functions [17].

Normal bladder function during filling/storage implies no significant rises in detrusor pressure (stability). Overactive detrusor function indicates the presence of involuntary contractions. If owing to neurologic disease, the term detrusor hyperreflexia is used; if not, the phenomenon is known as detrusor instability. Bladder sensation can be categorized only in qualitative terms as indicated. Bladder capacity and compliance (Δ volume/Δ pressure) are cystometric measurements. Normal urethral function during filling/storage indicates a positive urethral closure pressure (urethral pressure minus bladder pressure) even with increases in intra-abdominal pressure. Incompetent urethral function during filling storage implies urine leakage in the absence of a detrusor contraction.

This may be secondary to genuine stress incontinence, intrinsic sphincter dysfunction, or an involuntary fall in urethral pressure in the absence of a detrusor contraction.

During the voiding/emptying phase of micturition, normal detrusor activity implies voiding by a voluntarily initiated, sustained contraction that also can be suppressed voluntarily. An underactive detrusor defines a contraction of inadequate magnitude and/or duration to empty the bladder with a normal time span. An acontractile detrusor is the one that cannot be demonstrated to contract during urodynamic testing. Areflexia is defined as acontractility owing to an abnormality of neural control, implying the complete absence of centrally coordinated contraction. Normal urethral function during voiding indicates opening prior to micturition to allow bladder emptying. An obstructed urethra is one which contracts against a detrusor contraction or fails to open (nonrelaxation) with attempted micturition. Contraction may be owing to smooth or striated sphincter dyssynergia. Striated sphincter dyssynergia is a term that should be applied only when neurologic disease is present. A similar syndrome, though not associated to any neurologic disease, is called dysfunctional voiding. Mechanical obstruction is generally anatomical and caused by BPH, urethral or bladder neck stricture, scarring or compression, or, rarely, kinking of a portion of the urethra during straining.

Voiding dysfunction in a classic T-10 level paraplegic after spinal shock has passed would be classified as follows:

1. Storage phase: overactive hyperreflexic detrusor, absent sensation, low capacity, normal compliance, and normal urethral closure function
2. Voiding phase: overactive obstructive urethral function and normal detrusor activity (actually, hyperreflexic)

The voiding dysfunction of a stroke patient with urgency incontinence would most likely be classified during storage as overactive hyperreflexic detrusor, normal sensation, low capacity, normal compliance, and normal urethral closure function. During voiding, the dysfunction would be classified as normal detrusor activity and normal urethral function, assuming that no anatomic obstruction existed.

10.3.7 Functional System

Classification of voiding dysfunction can also be formulated on a simple functional basis, describing the dysfunction in terms of whether the deficit produced is primarily one of the filling/storage or emptying phases of micturition (Fig. 10.1) [1, 18].

This type of system was proposed initially by Quesada et al. [19] and is an excellent alternative when a particular dysfunction does not readily lend itself to a generally agreed upon classification elsewhere. This simple-minded scheme only assumes that, whatever their differences that might be reported, all "experts" would agree on the two-phase concept of micturition and upon the simple overall mechanisms underlying the normality of each phase. Storage failure results because of either bladder or outlet abnormalities or a combination. Bladder abnormalities include involuntary bladder contractions, low compliance, and hypersensitivity. The outlet abnormalities include only an intermittent or continuous decrease in outlet resistance.

Similarly, emptying failure can occur because of bladder or outlet abnormalities or a combination of the two. The bladder side includes inadequate bladder contractility, and the outlet side includes anatomic obstruction and sphincter(s) dyssynergia.

Failure in either category generally is not absolute, but more frequently relative. Such a functional system can easily be "expanded" and made more complicated by the inclusion of etiologic or specific urodynamic connotations. However, the simplified system is perfectly workable and avoids argument in those complex situations in which the exact etiology or urodynamic mechanism for a voiding dysfunction cannot be agreed upon.

Proper use of this system for a given voiding dysfunction obviously requires a reasonably accurate notion of what the urodynamic data show. However, an exact diagnosis is not required for treatment. It should be recognized that some patients do not only have a discrete storage or emptying failure, and the existence of combination deficits must be recognized to properly utilize this system of classification. One of the advantages of this functional classification is that it allows the individual the liberty of "playing" with the system to suit his or her preferences without an alteration in the basic concept of "keep it simple but accurate and informative." For instance, one could easily substitute "overactive or oversensitive bladder" and "outlet insufficiency" for "because of the bladder" and "because of the outlet" under "failure to store." One could choose to subcategorize the bladder reasons for overactivity in terms of neurogenic, myogenic, or anatomic etiologies and further subcategorize neurogenic in terms of increased afferent activity, decreased inhibitory control, increased sensitivity to efferent activity, and so forth. The system is flexible.

An additional advantage to the functional system is that the underlying concepts can be used repeatedly to simplify many areas in neuro-urology. One logical extension makes urodynamics become more readily understandable, whereas a different type of adaptation functions especially well as a "menu" for the categorization of all the types of treatment for voiding dysfunction.

The major problem with the functional system is that not every voiding dysfunction can be reduced or converted primarily to a failure of storage or emptying. Additionally, although the functional classification of therapy correlated with this scheme is entirely logical and complete, there is a danger of accepting an easy therapeutic solution and of thereby overlooking an etiology for a voiding dysfunction that is reversible at the primary level of causation. Non-neurogenic voiding dysfunctions, however, can be classified within this system, including those involving only the sensory aspect of micturition.

It is obvious that no type of classification system is perfect. Each one offers something to every clinician, although his or her level and type of trainings, interests, experiences, and prejudices regarding the accuracy and interpretation of urodynamic data will determine a system's usefulness. The ideal approach to a patient with voiding dysfunction continues to be a thorough neuro-urologic evaluation. If the clinician can classify a given patient's voiding dysfunction in each system or can understand why this cannot be done, there is enough working knowledge to proceed with treatment.

References

1. Wein AJ, Barrett DM. Voiding function and dysfunction: a logical and practical approach. Chicago: Year Book Medical Publishers; 1988.
2. Wein AJ. Pathophysiology and categorization of voiding dysfunction. In: Walsh PC, Retik AB, Vaughan Jr ED, Wein AJ, editors. Campbell's urology. 8th ed. Philadelphia: WB Saunders Co; 1998. p. 917–26.
3. Zderie SA, Levin RM, Wein AJ. Voiding function: relevant anatomy, physiology, pharmacology and molecular aspects. In: Gillenwater JY, Grayhack JT, Howards SS, Duckett Jr JW, editors. Adult and pediatric urology. Chicago: Year Book Medical Publishers; 1996. p. 1159–219.
4. Steers WD. Physiology and pharmacology of the bladder and urethra. In: Walsh PC, Retik AB, Vaughan Jr ED, Wein AJ, editors. Campbell's urology. 8th ed. Philadelphia: WB Saunders Co; 1998. p. 870–916.
5. DeLaneey JOL. Structural support of the urethra as it relates to stress urinary incontinence: the harnrnock hypothesis. Am J Obstet Gynecol. 1994;170:1713.
6. Panicker JN, Fowler CJ, Kessler TM. Lower urinary tract dysfunction in the neurological patient: clinical assessment and management. Lancet Neurol. 2015;14(7):720–32.
7. Kuhtz-Buschbeck JP, van der Horst C, Pott C, et al. Cortical representation of the urge to void: a functional magnetic resonance imaging study. J Urol. 2005;174:1477–81.
8. Panicker JN, de Sèze M, Fowler CJ. Rehabilitation in practice: neurogenic lower urinary tract dysfunction and its management. Clin Rehabil. 2010;24(2010):579–89.
9. Stoehrer M, Blok B, Castro-Diaz D, Chartier-Kastler E, Del Popolo G, Kramer G, Pannek J, Radziszewski P, Wyndaele JJ. EAU guidelines on neurogenic lower urinary tract dysfunction. Eur Urol. 2009;56:81–8.
10. Madersbacher H. The various types of neurogenic bladder dysfunction: an update of current therapeutic concepts. Paraplegia. 1990;28:217–29.
11. Bors E, Comarr AE. Neurological urology. Baltimore: University Park Press; 1971.
12. Hald T, Bradley WE. The urinary bladder: neurology and dynamics. Baltimore: Williams and Wilkins; 1982.
13. Markland C, Chou S, Westgate H, Bradley WE. Neuro-urologic evaluation of neurologic bladder dysfunction. Proc Annu Clin Spinal Cord Inj Conf. 1967;16:123–3.
14. Lapides J. Neurogenic bladder. Principles of treatment. Urol Clin North Am. 1974;1(1):81–97.
15. McLellan FC. The neurogenic bladder. Springfield: Charles Thomas Co; 1939. p. 57–70. 116-185.
16. Krane RJ, Siroky MB. Classification of voiding dysfunction: value of classification systems. In: Barrett DM, Wein AJ, editors. Controversies in neurourology. New York: Churchill Livingstone; 1984. p. 223–38.
17. Abrams P, Blaivas JG, Stanton SL, Andersen JT. The standardization of terminology of lower urinary tract function recommended by the International Continence Society. Intl Urogynecol J. 1990;1:45.
18. Wein AJ. Classification of neurogenic voiding dysfunction. J Urol. 1981;125:605.
19. Quesada EM, Seott FB, Cardus D. Functional classification of neurogenic bladder dysfunction. Arch Phys Med Rehabil. 1968;49:692.

Treatment of Chronic Pelvic Pain: Multidisciplinary Approach

11

Bart Morlion and Flaminia Coluzzi

Chronic pelvic pain (CPP) can be defined as intermittent or constant pain, perceived in structures related to the lower abdomen or pelvis of either men or women and recurring over a 6-month period. CPP has a major impact on health-related quality of life, work productivity and health care utilization.

Chronic pelvic pain syndrome (CPPS) is a subdivision of CPP, identified as a complex non-malignant pain syndrome, when no proven infection or other obvious local pathologies that may be accounted for the pain can be detected. CPPS is associated with negative cognitive, behavioural, sexual and emotional consequences as well as with symptoms of sexual, intestinal, perineal, gynaecological or lower urinary tract dysfunction.

CPPS may be focused on a single pelvic organ or affect two or more pelvic apparatuses and even be associated with systemic diseases, such as fibromyalgia and depression.

The challenge of CPPS raises from the diversity of potential etiological factors, the high number of possible anatomical source of pain as well as the potential assumption that chronic pain may be a disease itself rather than a symptom. The most common pathologies associated with CPP are presented in Table 11.1. The history and physical examination are often powerful diagnostic tools in CPPS. However, consultations with other specialists may be needed. A multidisciplinary approach is then often indicated in both the diagnostic and therapeutic phases.

B. Morlion
The Leuven Centre for Algology, University Hospitals Leuven, University of Leuven, Leuven, Belgium

Medical Faculty KU Leuven, Leuven, Belgium

F. Coluzzi (✉)
Department of Medico-Surgical Sciences and Biotechnologies, Unit of Anaesthesia, Intensive Care and Pain Medicine, Sapienza University of Rome, Rome, Italy
e-mail: flaminia.coluzzi@uniroma1.it

© Springer International Publishing Switzerland 2016
A. Carbone et al. (eds.), *Functional Urologic Surgery in Neurogenic and Oncologic Diseases*, Urodynamics, Neurourology and Pelvic Floor Dysfunctions, DOI 10.1007/978-3-319-29191-8_11

Table 11.1 Common diseases causing CPPS

Gynaecological	Urological	Gastrointestinal	Musculoskeletal	Neurologic	Sexual
Endometriosis	Painful bladder syndrome	Irritable bowel syndrome	Pelvic floor dysfunction	Post-herpetic neuralgia	Dyspareunia
Adenomyosis	Chronic prostatitis	Inflammatory bowel disease	Myofascial pain syndrome	Incisional neuroma	Sexual dysfunction
Pelvic congestion syndrome	Acute recurrent cystitis	Chronic constipation	Adhesions	Visceral hyperalgesia	
Adhesion	Post-radiation cystitis	Colon malignancy	Fibromyalgia	Pudendal neuralgia	
Ovarian remnant syndrome	Chronic urinary tract infections	Colitis	Muscular sprains (rectus muscle)	Entrapment neuropathy	
Pelvic inflammatory disease	Uninhibited bladder contraction	Hernia	Pyriformis syndrome		
Malignancy	Urolithiasis	Diverticular disease	Chronic coccygeal pain		
Cervical stenosis	Urethral diverticulum	Diarrhoea	Low back pain		
Adnexal cyst	Urethral caruncle				
Symptomatic pelvic relaxation	Urethral syndrome				
Salpingitis	Malignancy				
Prostatitis					

11.1 Common Diseases Causing CPPS

11.1.1 Painful Bladder Syndrome

The main urological disease causing CPPS is the painful bladder syndrome (PBS), previously called interstitial cystitis (IC), diagnosed by the presence of the classic triad: urinary urgency and frequency, pelvic pain and mucosal haemorrhages with cystoscopic hydrodistension, in the absence of urinary infection or other pathologies, such as bladder tumours or radiation-induced cystitis.

PBS is more common among women than men. Traditionally, voiding frequency is every 2 h or less, without incontinence. Pelvic pain is referred as pressure or discomfort to the bladder and usually occurs at the end of voiding or at full bladder. Urinalysis and urine culture may be useful for the exclusion of infections. Cystoscopic evaluation is not mandatory for diagnosis, since a number of false positives may occur. However, mucosal haemorrhages, called glomerulations, reduced bladder capacity, linear cracking and Hunner ulcer are considered typical signs of disease. Cystoscopy may be particularly painful in these patients; therefore, analgosedation and general or spinal anaesthesia may be needed [1].

11.1.2 Chronic Prostatitis

Chronic prostatitis (CP) is a highly prevalent condition affecting men, with severe effects in terms of quality of life. CP can be bacterial (acute or chronic), inflammatory (symptomatic or asymptomatic) or noninflammatory, characterized by chronic pelvic pain and voiding symptoms, with no evidence of bacterial infection nor inflammation. CPPS is localized to the prostate, perineum or urethra, but its aetiology is still poorly understood. CP/CPPS may be caused by antibiotic-resistant microorganisms, urethral obstruction, reflux of urine in the prostatic ducts, immune dysregulation, pudendal nerve entrapment, myofascial or pelvic floor muscles pain. Neuropathic pain may play an important role in CP/CPPS, and it should be considered as a target of the analgesic treatment [1].

11.1.3 Endometriosis

Endometriosis is the most common cause of CPPS in women and is caused by ectopic endometrial tissue located outside of the uterus. The prevalence in women of reproductive age worldwide is 10–15 % and over 30 % among women with CPPS. The symptoms typically recur in a cyclic fashion, and their exacerbation may also occur around menstruation. Ninety percent of women with endometriosis-related CPPS have dysmenorrhoea and 40 % have dyspareunia. Clinical diagnosis, mainly based on the history (CPPS, dysmenorrhoea, infertility and adnexal masses) of the patient, is accurate in about 80 % of the cases. Histologic confirmation can be assessed on a tissue biopsy sample obtained from an extrauterine location showing endometrial glands. Hormonal treatment (oral contraceptive pills, progestins, androgens and gonadotropin-releasing hormone agonists), surgery and excision of endometrial implants are all appropriate options to manage pain associated with endometriosis [2].

11.1.4 Irritable Bowel Syndrome

Irritable bowel syndrome (IBS) is a common gastrointestinal (GI) functional disorder that affects the large intestine, characterized by signs and symptoms of constipation, diarrhoea, bloating, abdominal cramping and pain. Its prevalence, as defined by the Rome II or III criteria, ranges from 4.3 to 13.5 %. The three elements of pathophysiology of IBS are altered GI motility, visceral hyperalgesia and psychological factors. Colonic dysmotility in IBS has been associated to generalized smooth muscle hyperresponsiveness, leading often to urinary symptoms. In some patients microscopic inflammation and alteration of the intestinal microbiota have been observed. Causes are still unclear, but include previous enteric infections, neuro-hormonal interaction, intestinal permeability and dietary intolerance [3]. Treatment options include non-pharmacological (exercise, sleep, probiotics, gluten-free diet) and pharmacological approaches (peripheral μ-opioid receptor agonist loperamide, antispasmodic agents, antidepressants, serotonin 5-HT3 antagonists and the gut-specific antibiotic rifaximin) [4].

11.1.5 Adhesions

Peritoneal adhesions are a common consequence of any intra-abdominal inflammatory process, such as pelvic inflammatory disease (PID) and diverticulitis. Up to 90 % of patients after surgery develop intra-abdominal adhesions. Adhesiolysis for peritubular and periovarian adhesions, and enterolysis for bowel adhesions, may be an adequate surgical approach to CPPS due to adhesions [5].

11.2   Chronic Pelvic Pain Syndrome: Pathophysiology

11.2.1 Central Sensitization

Chronic pelvic pain reflects a state of excitability of central nociceptive circuits, called central sensitization. The result of central sensitization is visceral hypersensitivity, with enhanced perception of visceral stimuli and altered autonomic regulation of the gut.

Central sensitization can be defined as an amplification of neural signalling within the central nervous system (CNS) that elicits pain hypersensitivity. Central sensitization has been hypothesized to contribute to a number of chronic pain syndromes, including the painful bladder syndrome, chronic prostatitis, endometriosis and vulvodynia. When a central amplification occurs, the pain response to both non-noxious and noxious stimuli is enhanced in amplitude, duration and spatial extent, leading to hyperalgesia and allodynia. Hyperalgesia means an increased response to a painful stimulus. Allodynia refers to a painful response to a normally innocuous stimulus. Spontaneous positive sensations like paraesthesia and dysaesthesia, paroxysmal pain and ongoing superficial pain may also occur. Hyperalgesia, allodynia and other positive symptoms are typical clinical manifestations of chronic "neuropathic pain", arising as a direct consequence of a lesion or disease affecting the somatosensory system. Neuropathic pain is the expression of maladaptive plasticity within the nociceptive system [6].

"Nociceptive pain" is an adaptive response to noxious stimulus, where primary afferent nociceptive Aδ and C fibres terminate in the spinal dorsal horn at two types of neurons: spinal projection neurons, which innervate higher neuronal centres including the thalamus, and interneurons with various functions.

Neuroplasticity in the dorsal horn represents the main pathological change occurring during central sensitization and causing chronic neuropathic pain. Several maladaptive phenomena explain the hyperexcitability state: (1) pronociceptive facilitation at the spinal dorsal horn, caused by the activation of N-methyl-D-aspartate (NMDA) receptor by glutamate, the major excitatory transmitter; (2) disinhibition of nociception at the spinal inhibitory network; and (3) central cortical reorganization of the primary somatosensory projection area [7].

Peripheral sensitization also occurs as a result of the release of inflammatory agents (e.g. adenosines, bradykinins, cytokines, amino acids, histamines, nerve growth factors and prostaglandins).

11.2.2 Crosstalk

The precise mechanism underlying pelvic pain remains still unclear. However, it is well known that pelvic organs and structures communicate through nerve connections or reflexes. This phenomenon, named neural crosstalk, may play a role in the overlap of CPP disorders [8]. Up to 40 % of patients diagnosed with IC also have symptoms for IBS and over 25 % have also vulvodynia. Cross-sensitization in the pelvis is considered as one of the factors contributing to CPPS: the transmission of noxious stimuli from a diseased pelvic organ to an adjacent normal structure results in the occurrence of functional and rarely structural changes in the latter. Experimental evidence shows that colorectal distension inhibits urination (colon-to-bladder cross inhibition) and, during urination, colonic motor activity is inhibited (bladder-to-colon cross inhibition) [9]. Similarly, PBS/CPPS, with documented inflammation and increased vascular permeability of the bladder, may be alleviated by 2 % lidocaine instillation into either the bladder or the colon, even though colon histology was normal. These data explain why dietary modification may impact pelvic pain symptoms. Viscerovisceral interactions and reflexes between gastrointestinal, urinary and reproductive systems are thought to underlie pelvic organ cross-sensitization, by three different interconnected neural pathways: (1)

convergence of sensory neural pathways within a dorsal root ganglion (DRG), from a diseased pelvic organ to a normal adjacent structure; (2) convergence of afferent information in the spinal cord; and (3) convergence of afferent inputs from two different pelvic organs in the brain.

11.2.3 Neurogenic Inflammation

Neurogenic inflammation plays a role in a variety of disorders, including CPPS. Neurogenic inflammation is caused by the release of substance P and calcitonin gene-related peptide (CGRP) from sensory nerves, which stimulates vasodilation, microvascular plasma extravasation and mast cell degranulation. There is an interaction between the neurogenic inflammation in the brain, leading to increased permeability of the blood-brain barrier (BBB), and classical inflammation: many of the factors within each process may initiate or potentiate the other cascade.

11.3 Pharmacological Management of CPPS

The targets of treatment for chronic pelvic pain, in order of priority, are (1) to manage underlying disease, (2) to reduce pain intensity, (3) to minimize side effects and (4) to optimize patient function and quality of life [10].

Specific pathological components of the pelvic pain and comorbidities may require referral to a specialist. A multidisciplinary team approach is essential. Women suffering from endometriosis require gynaecological evaluation and hormonal treatment (hormonal contraceptives, progestagens, anti-progestagens or GnRH agonists). Patients with IBS may obtain benefits from dietary modifications, probiotics and a gastroenterological consultation. Urologists should be involved in the management of patients suffering from prostate pain syndrome, in which alpha-blockers (terazosin, alfuzosin, doxazosin, tamsulosin and silodosin), antibiotic therapy and 5-alpha-reductase inhibitors (finasteride) can be prescribed. Similarly, they have a key role in the management of patients with PBS.

General treatment of CPPS requires an early multimodal treatment with symptomatic analgesics to reduce the severity of pain. The neuropathic component of pain should be detected by using appropriate tools, such as the questionnaire DN4. In managing chronic pain, mechanism-oriented treatment is supposed to be more effective than intensity-based analgesic selection. Adjuvants, such as antidepressants and anticonvulsants, play a major role in the management of neuropathic pain syndromes. Opioids represent a valid alternative for moderate-to-severe chronic pain, when long-term use of analgesic is required.

The most recent guidelines on chronic pelvic pain are available from the Royal College of Obstetricians and Gynaecologists (NICE accredited 2012) [11], the British Pain Society (2014) [12] and the European Association of Urology (2012) [13].

11.3.1 Nonsteroidal Anti-inflammatory Drugs (NSAIDs) and Paracetamol

Anti-inflammatory analgesics, such as NSAIDs, inhibit the enzyme cyclooxygenase (COX) and also have a peripheral effect. They are indicated in CPPS, when the inflammatory component is prevalent, such as in dysmenorrhoea. Conversely, their efficacy is weak in chronic pain syndromes, where the central sensitization is relevant, such as in endometriosis. Moreover, their use is limited by poor tolerability profile in the gastrointestinal and cardiovascular systems.

Paracetamol is a central analgesic with antipyretic activity. Its use is recommended at the maximal daily dose of 4 g. Paracetamol can be used in fixed association with opioids, such as codeine, tramadol and oxycodone. Despite its use dates back over 100 years, the exact mechanism of analgesic action of paracetamol is still poorly understood. Recent studies suggest a role for the serotoninergic inhibitory descending system and for the endocannabinoid system.

11.3.2 Antidepressant Drugs

The analgesic properties of antidepressant drugs have been reported since the 1960s and have been shown to be independent from their antidepressant activity. Antidepressants are widely used for the treatment of chronic pain, specifically in neuropathic pain syndromes. Tricyclic antidepressants (TCAs), such as amitriptyline (up to 150 mg daily), still represent the gold standard of treatment, because they have the lowest number needed to treat (NNT, number of patients to be treated to obtain at least one patient with 50 % pain relief) compared with other adjuvants. However, their poor tolerability profile significantly limited their clinical use in fewer specific conditions. Many side effects may be related to the antimuscarinic properties of the TCAs. The most common side effects of tricyclic antidepressants include dry mouth, blurred vision, constipation, urinary retention, drowsiness, increased appetite leading to weight gain, hypotension and increased sweating. Special caution is needed for patients with heart rate abnormalities; a 12-lead electrocardiogram (ECG) is required before starting treatment. Sinus tachycardia, prolonged QTc duration, prolonged PR interval, AV block and non-specific ST changes can occur in TCA overdose.

Selective serotonin reuptake inhibitors (SSRIs), such as sertraline, have been shown to be less effective as analgesics; therefore their use is not recommended in chronic pain management. However they can be used as antidepressants to manage depression, as a comorbidity of chronic pain. Depressive symptoms are particularly common in women suffering from CPPS.

A new class of antidepressants, named serotonin and noradrenaline reuptake inhibitors (SNRIs), are more selective than TCAs and have a balanced reuptake inhibition of both neurotransmitters. Compared with the traditional TCAs, they do not have the adverse events due to the activity of TCAs on histamine, acetylcholine and dopamine. This new class includes venlafaxine (37.5–75 mg daily) and dulox-etine (30–60 mg daily).

The main problem in evaluating the efficacy of antidepressants in chronic uro-logical pelvic pain is the heterogeneity of the clinical studies, due to different con-founding factors: (1) most of the studies are uncontrolled prospective case series, (2) methodological bias and low-quality clinical trials and (3) inconsistency of the classification of chronic pelvic pain syndrome [14].

However, despite these limitations, antidepressants may have a role in managing urological CPP.

11.3.3 Gabapentinoids

Among anticonvulsant drugs, gabapentinoids (gabapentin and pregabalin) are the most commonly used for chronic pain management. Their analgesic activity is mediated by the ability to selectively bind to the alpha-2-delta subunit of voltage-gated calcium channel. Therefore, gabapentinoids reduce the influx of calcium into the cell, thereby reducing the synaptic release of neurotransmitters, such as gluta-mate, norepinephrine and substance P. Pregabalin has the same biologic activity of gabapentin, but improved pharmacokinetic profile (i.e. higher potency, increased oral bioavailability, linear pharmacokinetics). Dosage adjustments are required for patients suffering from renal dysfunction.

Both gabapentinoids and antidepressants are recommended in monotherapy as first-line treatment of neuropathic pain. When the monotherapy does not obtain adequate analgesia, it is recommended to switch or to add to the alternative class (i.e. if a patient is not adequately managed with antidepressants in monotherapy, it is possible to switch to a gabapentinoid or to add it in a poly-pharmacological approach). The most common adverse events of gabapentinoids are dizziness and sedation. In order to minimize side effects, the daily dose should be slowly increased up to a maximum dose of 3,600 mg gabapentin and 600 mg pregabalin.

Although anticonvulsants are used widely in chronic pain, surprisingly few trials showed analgesic effectiveness in CPPS. Hence, recommendations were made according to non-specific data, extrapolated from references on neuropathic pain regardless of the CPP mechanisms.

11.3.4 Opioids

Opioids are the mainstay of analgesic treatment for severe chronic pain. They are usually classified as weak (codeine, tramadol, transdermal buprenorphine) and strong (morphine, oxycodone, hydrocodone, hydromorphone, transdermal fen-tanyl). Extended-release formulations are preferred in chronic pain management, while rapid-onset opioids (fentanyl formulations with fast onset of action and short half-life) are recommended for breakthrough pain in the cancer setting.

The effectiveness of opioids in neuropathic pain is still under discussion, because the available clinical trials have a number of limitations: few patients, short-term observations (up to 12 weeks) and limited randomized controlled trials. Moreover, preclinical studies showed that mu-opioid receptors are downregulated in neuropathic pain animal models (sciatic nerve ligation), while noradrenergic sprouting has been observed in the dorsal horn of these animals. Noradrenergic tone seems to play a key role in regulating neuropathic pain progression. Hence, among opioids, tapentadol (the first drug of a new pharmacological class named mu-opioid receptor agonist/noradrenaline reuptake inhibitors (MOR/NRI)) is recommended as first choice in patients suffering from chronic pain with a neuropathic component. Its lower affinity for MOR (50 times lower than morphine) makes tapentadol significantly more tolerable than traditional opioids, such as oxycodone. Nausea and vomiting are common effects in the first phases of opioid treatment, but usually disappear within 7–10 days, due to the development of tolerance. Instead, the most common and persistent side effect during chronic treatment is opioid-induced constipation (OIC), due to the activity of MOR dislocated in the myenteric and submucosal plexus of the gastrointestinal (GI) tract. Tapentadol significantly reduced OIC compared with oxycodone. Similarly, the association oxycodone/naloxone, at the ratio 2:1, significantly improved bowel dysfunction in patients with chronic pain. When administrated by the oral route, the bioavailability of the MOR antagonist naloxone is about 2 %, due to a wide first-pass hepatic metabolism; therefore its activity is limited to the GI tract, without affecting the systemic analgesia of oxycodone.

These new opioid formulations were specifically studied to improve the side effect profile of opioids, in order to improve patient adherence to chronic pain treatment.

When starting opioids for chronic non-cancer pain management, some essential roles should be followed: (1) correct diagnosis, (2) establish treatment goals, (3) titrate the opioid to the minimal effective dose, (4) prefer oral administration, (5) use extended-release formulations to obtain a stable plasma concentration, (6) prevent or manage side effects, (7) re-evaluate the patient after a trial of treatment and (8) consider the potential for physical dependency and addiction.

11.3.5 N-Palmitoyl-Ethanolamine (PEA)

N-palmitoyl-ethanolamine (PEA) is an endogenous fatty acid amide, well known as an important analgesic, anti-inflammatory and neuroprotective mediator, acting at several molecular targets in both central and sensory nervous systems. PEA acts by downregulating mast cell degranulation and by enhancing the anti-inflammatory and antinociceptive effects exerted by the endocannabinoid, anandamide. When stimulated, mast cells release a number of mediators that initiate an inflammatory response and can also regulate the activity of other immune cells, including central microglia.

Glial cell activation and neuroinflammation are known to be one of the underlying causes of chronic pain syndromes, including CPPS (interstitial cystitis, endometriosis and vulvodynia).

Among nutraceuticals, the association of micronized PEA-transpolydatin has been shown to be effective on chronic pelvic pain associated with endometriosis, by reducing mast cell activation in endometriotic lesions [15].

11.3.6 Botulinum A Toxin (BTX-A)

Botulinum A toxin (BTX-A) is an inhibitor of acetylcholine release at the neuromuscular junction and has a paralyzing effect on striated muscles. BTX-A may have an antinociceptive effect on bladder afferent pathways; however limited data exist on the effectiveness of BTX-A injection into the detrusor or trigone. BTX-A can be used for the treatment of chronic pelvic pain associated with spasm of the levator ani muscles and to reduce the resting pressure in the pelvic floor muscles.

11.4 Interventional Techniques for CPPS

Afferent information from pelvic viscera travels to DRGs and further to the spinal dorsal horn mainly via hypogastric, splanchnic, pelvic and pudendal nerves. These nerves convey sensory information from major pelvic organs: the colon, rectum, urinary bladder and uterus. Nerve blocks can be used to manage CPPS; however they rarely provide long-term analgesia and require sequential injections with local anaesthetics. The duration of their analgesic effect and potential complications (including X-ray exposure) should be considered. Superior hypogastric plexus (SHP) blocks are useful for relieving CPP associated with PBS, IBS, endometriosis, adhesions and chronic pain related to the bladder, prostate, testes, uterus, ovaries, vagina, colon and rectum. SHP blocks can be used for either diagnostic or therapeutic purposes. Ganglion impar block is indicated for perineal pain from the rectum, anus, distal urethra, vulva and distal third of the vagina.

Neurolytic blocks, such as SHP block, are used in the management of pelvic pain related to cancers. Non-surgical neurolysis can be performed with chemicals (alcohol or phenol), cryoablation or thermocoagulation.

Neuromodulation of the sacral nerves has been used for treating visceral pelvic pain, such as PBS. Appropriate diagnosis is a key factor for success. An electrode is placed through the transforaminal approach into the S3 or S4 foramen in the area of the nerve roots. Stimulation has to be perceived in the site of perceived pain. After a trial of spinal cord stimulation (SCS), conducted to confirm the effectiveness in CPP, if the patient obtains adequate analgesia, a permanent stimulator implantation is performed.

Transcutaneous electrical nerve stimulation (TENS) is widely used; however evidence is still poor.

11.5   Non-pharmacological Management of CPPS

Psychological distress is common in pelvic pain, particularly in women. Sexual abuse should be assessed as possible contributory factors in CPPS. Psychological intervention may significantly improve pain relief as well as mood and quality of life.

The physiotherapist is part of the pain management team. Physical therapies are used for the overactivity of the pelvic floor muscle. Patients should learn how to relax the muscles when the pain starts. Similarly, biofeedback and electrostimulation can be useful in the treatment of pelvic floor muscle pain.

11.6   Multimodal and Multidisciplinary Approach to CPPS

The latest paradigm shift in the thinking about CPPS parallels the evolution in concepts of chronic pain in general.

The biopsychosocial model of chronic pain recognizes chronic pain as a combination of physical dysfunction, beliefs, coping strategies, distress, illness behaviour and social interactions. Since the introduction of the biopsychosocial model, treatment of chronic pain has become multimodal and multidisciplinary, with the aim of maximizing pain reduction, quality of life, independence and mobility.

Similarly, the CPPS is now considered as a biopsychosocial illness involving physical, behavioural, occupational and socioeconomic factors. More importantly, even if an initial injury in an anatomical structure can be identified, the pain experience and disability of an individual will be determined by an array of psychosocial factors, including previous pain experiences, beliefs and fears about CLBP, general and psychosocial health, job satisfaction, economic status, education, ongoing litigation, compensation claims and social well-being. This knowledge is often ignored, and many diagnostic procedures and therapies that are focused solely on peripheral anatomical structures in the pelvis continue to be offered with a high risk for iatrogenic worsening of the complaints.

References

1. Strauss AC, Dimitrakov JD. New treatments for chronic prostatitis/chronic pelvic pain syndrome. Nat Rev Urol. 2010;7(3):127–35.
2. Ahn SH, Monsanto SP, Miller C, Singh SS, Thomas R, Tayade C. Pathophysiology and immune dysfunction in endometriosis. Biomed Res Int. 2015;2015:795976.
3. Lacy BE, Chey WD, Lembo AJ. New and emerging treatment options for irritable bowel syndrome. Gastroenterol Hepatol (N Y). 2015;11(4 Suppl 2):1–19.
4. Baranowski AP. Chronic pelvic pain. Best Pract Res Clin Gastroenterol. 2009;23:593–610.
5. Holloran-Schwartz MB. Surgical evaluation and treatment of the patient with chronic pelvic pain. Obstet Gynecol Clin N Am. 2014;41(3):357–69.
6. Woolf CJ. Central sensitization: implications for the diagnosis and treatment of pain. Pain. 2011;152:S2–15.

7. Nickel FT, Seifert F, Lanz S, Maihöfner C. Mechanisms of neuropathic pain. Eur Neuropsychopharmacol. 2012;22:81–91.
8. Rudick CN, Chen MC, Mongiu AK, Klumpp DJ. Organ cross talk modulates pelvic pain. Am J Physiol Regul Integr Comp Physiol. 2007;293(3):R1191–8.
9. Malykina AP. Neural mechanism of pelvic organ cross-sensitization. Neuroscience. 2007;149:660–72.
10. Smith BH, Lee J, Price C, Baranowski AP. Neuropathic pain: a pathway for care developed by the British Pain Society. Br J Anaesth. 2013;11:73–9.
11. RCOG. The initial management of chronic pelvic pain. Ed2 green top 41. London: Royal College of Obstetricians and Gynaecologists; 2012.
12. Baranowski AP, Lee J, Price C, Hughes J. Pelvic pain: a pathway for care developed for both men and women by the British Pain Society. Br J Anaesth. 2014;112(3):452–9.
13. Engeler D, Baranowski AP, Elneil S, et al. EAU guidelines on chronic pelvic pain. Available from http://www.uroweb.org/guidelines/online-guidelines/. Accessed Sept 2015.
14. Papandreou C, Skapinakis P, Giannakis D, Sofikitis N, Mavreas V. Antidepressant drugs for chronic urological pelvic pain: an evidence-based review. Adv Urol. 2009;2009:797031.
15. Indraccolo U, Barbieri F. Effect of palmitoylethanolamide-polydatin combination on chronic pelvic pain associated with endometriosis: preliminary observations. Eur J Obstet Gynecol Reprod Biol. 2010;150(1):76–9.

Bladder Outlet Obstruction in Neurogenic Patients: When is Surgery Mandatory?

12

Giovanni Palleschi and Yazan Al Salhi

In patients with neurogenic vesico-sphincteric disease, bladder outlet obstruction (BOO) may further increase the risk of complications to the lower and upper urinary tract, such as high post-voiding residual urine, urinary infections, bladder stones formation, vesicoureteral reflux, and ureterohydronephrosis. These complications, if not treated, can inexorably lead to a severe damage of renal function, thus forcing patients to dialysis. The main cause of BOO in patients with neurogenic bladder (NB) has a functional origin represented by detrusor sphincter dyssynergia (DSD); however, it has to be considered that also an organic obstruction can develop in these subjects, especially in men. Furthermore, in some patients, both conditions may coexist. Therefore, only a correct diagnostic approach, based on a thorough knowledge and understanding of the pathophysiologic mechanisms involved in these conditions, may contribute to establish the adequate treatment and prevent potential iatrogenic complications. According to the International Consultation on Incontinence [1] and the European Association of Urology Guidelines [2], first-line therapeutic options of BOO in NB are represented by conservative approaches. Lifestyle interventions, alpha-1-adrenergic blockers, intermittent catheterization, and external specific devices (i.e., pessary in case of pelvic organ prolapse) have to be preferred until patient's QoL and therapeutic goals are maintained. When these treatments fail and cannot avoid the risk of the abovementioned severe complications to the urinary tract or when they do not achieve patient's satisfaction, surgery may become necessary.

G. Palleschi (✉) • Y. Al Salhi
Urology Unit, Department of Medico-Surgical Sciences and Biotechnologies,
Sapienza University of Rome, Latina, Italy
e-mail: giovanni.palleschi@uniroma1.it

© Springer International Publishing Switzerland 2016
A. Carbone et al. (eds.), *Functional Urologic Surgery in Neurogenic and Oncologic Diseases*, Urodynamics, Neurourology and Pelvic Floor Dysfunctions, DOI 10.1007/978-3-319-29191-8_12

12.1   Surgical Management of Detrusor Sphincter Dyssynergia (DSD)

The most common cause of functional BOO in patients with NB is represented by DSD. In this condition, a detrusor contraction occurs simultaneously with an inappropriate contraction of the urethral striated muscle, the periurethral striated muscle, or both, thus blocking the bladder outlet [3]. Normal micturition requires a synergic action between the detrusor muscle (smooth muscle) and the external urethral sphincter (striated muscle). To allow the bladder voiding phase, the external urethral sphincter relaxes, followed by a detrusor contraction; this synergic action is controlled by the pontine micturition center [4]. Disruption of the pathways between the pontine micturition center and the caudal part of the spinal cord often results in DSD. As a consequence, bladder emptying is poor, and it is exerted under high pressures with a risk of various consequences: high post-voiding residue, recurrent urinary infections, vesicoureteral reflux, and hydronephrosis. DSD usually develops in patients suffering from spinal cord lesions, above the sacral region. Presence and severity of DSD can be detected by urodynamic or videourodynamic investigation combined with striated sphincter needle electromyography. These diagnostic tests should also be periodically repeated during the follow-up of patients to check the effects of treatment and to verify that the clinic-functional conditions are stable. Different surgical therapies have been proposed and used for the treatment of DSD. For this reason, in 2014, Utomo et al. produced a Cochrane review with the aim to assess the effectiveness of different surgical approaches used to cure functional BOO in adults with NB [5]. Analyzing data from literature, the authors of the Cochrane review evaluated all the therapeutic options to treat DSD and provided the following reports:

1. *Sphincterotomy*: external sphincterotomy represents the transurethral treatment of the sphincter hypertonicity. It may be performed by an electrocautery or by laser energy. The goal of this treatment is to reduce the intravesical voiding pressure and to lower the detrusor leak point pressure. In some patients, a degree of continence can be saved if bladder neck function is preserved. The main reported complications are represented by postoperative bleeding, erectile dysfunction, urine extravasation, urethral stricture, and urinary fistula. However, it is reported that this treatment can provide an extended period of satisfactory bladder emptying [6].
2. *Urethral stents*: the urethral stents are mechanical devices (temporary or permanent) that can be placed in the urethra aiming to keep open the external urethral sphincter and thereby lower the detrusor leak point pressure. The first application of an urethral stent to treat DSD was by Shaw in 1990 [7], and then followers reported successful experiences with long-term clinical benefit and safety associated with improvement in maximum detrusor pressure and post-void residual urine volume, unchanged bladder capacity, and reduced hydronephrosis [8].
3. *Urethral balloon dilatation*: the first experience using balloon dilatation of the external urethral sphincter was reported by Chancellor in 1992 [9]. This device

(a balloon made by synthetic material) is placed under fluoroscopic guidance in the urethra at the site of the striated sphincter, and it is inflated to a diameter of 90 French under a pressure of 3 or 4 atmosphere for 10 min. Data reported by Chancellor showed effectiveness of this approach if compared with sphincterotomy [10]; McFarlane, after a personal experience, did not recommend this treatment due to a lack of real efficacy [11].

4. *Intraurethral botulinum A toxin (BTX A) injection*: BTX A is a neurotoxic protein produced by the bacterium *Clostridium botulinum*. This neurotoxin is responsible for an inhibition of the acetylcholine release at the neuromuscular junction inducing a muscle relaxation. BTX A is widely used in medicine to treat various pathological conditions, including NB dysfunction as detrusor overactivity. The first use of BTX A to treat DSD was reported by Dykstra in 1988 [12]; no many studies of high scientific value followed this experience. Schurch in 1996 reported favorable outcomes up to 3 months for the first BTX A treatment and a cumulative efficacy lasting 9–13 months [13].

5. *Intrathecal baclofen*: baclofen is a drug effective on skeletal muscle spasticity; it activates the gamma-aminobutyric acid-B receptors normalizing and decreasing interneuron and motor neuron activity in the spinal cord. Patients can receive a continuous intradural administration of baclofen by an implanted pump. This approach obviously reduces the risk of systemic side effects. Steers in 1992 reported interesting results showing 40% decrease of DSD in patients receiving baclofen for severe spasticity secondary to spinal cord injury [14]. Myazzato et al. provided the experimental evidence of the effect of baclofen on DSD showing a decrease of intravesical pressures in NB rats after spinal cord transection [15].

6. *Pudendal nerve block*: blocking the pudendal nerve (which contains motor axons to the external urethral sphincter), the activity of the external urethral sphincter is reduced. There are some experiences in literature regarding the use of phenol solution (administered by transcutaneous approach) to determine a neurolysis of pudendal nerve and treat DSD. Despite some favorable outcomes reported by various authors [15–17], some others reported that the duration of the effect is unpredictable.

7. *Suprapubic catheterization*: the insertion of an indwelling suprapubic catheter represents the most simple form of urinary diversion and some patients may need it. However, it has to be remarked that the use of an indwelling catheter is always associated with an increased risk of urinary infections, stones, erosions, bladder carcinoma (especially squamous subtype), even if the damage to the urethra is lower with a suprapubic device.

Basing on the Cochrane's authors report, there is no robust evidence in favor of any surgical treatment option for DSD treatment because of the limited availability of high-quality trials. Furthermore, the studies reported in literature are characterized by high variability of therapeutical approaches, small size of the cohorts involved, and too short duration of protocols. However, as an implication for clinical practice, this review showed an evidence of limited quality that BTX A injections improve the voided urine volume, lower the detrusor pressure, and decrease post-void residual volume. As a further consideration, a very important lack of all these studies is the absence of a standardized quality of life (QoL) assessment as a clinical outcome, and this bias is quite worrying, considering that medical success does not necessarily correspond with the emotional judgment reported by the patient.

12.2   Surgical Treatment in NB Patients with BOO Secondary to Benign Prostatic Hyperplasia (BPH)

There is still controversy regarding the use of surgical approaches to manage BOO secondary to BPH in patients with NB due to the potential increased risk of postoperative complications, mainly urinary incontinence. The lack of a common clinical and scientific point of view on this topic is mainly related to the scarce number of publications available in literature. Generally, patients who do not suffer from a peripheral denervation involving the pudendal nerve should not have negative consequences (especially stress urinary incontinence) from a prostatic surgery and might benefit from BOO removal. BPH is a progressive disease, and when medical treatment is unsuccessful, it can be responsible of recurrent infections, hematuria, and stone formation, especially in patients with neurogenic voiding dysfunction, but even more in those who practice self-intermittent catheterization. In all these situations, surgery could become mandatory. Today there are mini-invasive treatments which allow to reduce the risk of intra- and postoperative complications in NB patients with BOO, such as the use of urethral stents or similar devices which aim to dilate the prostatic urethra. However, there are still no data in literature which show the outcomes of these approaches in large cohorts and with an acceptable follow-up; therefore, a conclusive statement is not possible in this textbook. Literature provides few data from studies with limited case series regarding BPH surgical treatment in NB patients. Koyanagi et al. in 1987 reported their experience with radical transurethral resection of the prostate (TURP) performed on 89 male spinal cord injury subjects suffering from DSD and BOO [18]. Basing on postoperative urodynamic and striated sphincter electromyography, they described 90 % of success characterized by a reduced DSD, an increase of vesical compliance and a reduction in detrusor hyperreflexia. The authors reported also a 14 % recurrence rate of DSD with time. These results suggest an effect on the distal sphincteric area by the adrenergic system in the genesis of DSD. In fact, it is suggested that TURP exerts this effect via a surgical sympathectomy, while continence is preserved by the activity of the untouched external urethral sphincter. More data are available from literature regarding the treatment of BOO secondary to BPH in patients with Parkinson's disease (PD) [19]. PD is a common movement disorder (tremor at rest, rigidity, and gait difficulty) associated with the degeneration of dopaminergic neurons in the substantia nigra [20]. The fact that PD is the second most common degenerative neurological condition after Alzheimer's disease represents the main reason that explains the interest of neurologists and urologists in standardizing the approach of urinary disorders in these subjects, including BPH treatment [21].

Moreover, both PD and BPH are common in late middle-aged men; thus, their concurrence is probable. Lower urinary tract symptoms secondary to BPH such as weak urinary flow, urinary frequency, urinary urgency, and nocturia are common also in PD individuals, and considering that PD onset is insidious, clinicians could misdiagnose the two conditions. History and physical examination (general, urological, neurological) may induce the suspicious of neurogenicity of some symptoms (as intense urinary urgency, urgency urinary incontinence, stress urinary incontinence, or sexual dysfunctions). In these cases, the contribute of neurophysiological tests and of urodynamic or videourodynamic assessment with striated urethral sphincter electromyography can lead to a correct diagnostic evaluation allowing to avoid surgery in patients with risk of severe complications. These considerations are of utmost importance also because some neurogenic disorders may express lower urinary tract symptoms some years before the onset of the neurologic signs and could not be recognized if a rigorous diagnostic algorithm is not adopted. Patients with multisystemic atrophy (MSA), even sharing many PD like symptoms, can show urinary alterations since several years before the neurogenic onset [22]. Furthermore, MSA is a more severe, rapidly progressive, multisystemic, and fatal disease, and therefore, surgical treatment of BOO in these subjects results contraindicated for the certain development of severe complications. The clinical, urodynamic, and neurophysiological findings that allow to distinguish PD and MSA patients have been reported in literature and represent a concrete contribute for urologists and neurologists in the evaluation of these patients [23]. Under a clinical point of view, early symptoms onset, troublesome incontinence, and even earlier erectile dysfunction in men are regarded as warning signs of MSA [24]. From a neurophysiological point of view, the most important predictor of MSA is the neurogenic change of sphincter electromyography, which is rarely seen in patients with PD [25]. Another predictor of MSA is an open bladder neck at the start of bladder filling without accompanying DO, found in about 50 % of patients with MSA but not in PD patients. This finding indicates internal sphincter denervation [26].

Basing on the evidence of urodynamic and neurophysiologic findings reported in literature, it can be concluded that men with a definitive diagnosis of PD and coincidental BPH could be considered for appropriate surgery. Nowadays PD is no longer to be considered a contraindication for prostate surgery, and preoperative investigations, including urodynamic assessment, should be used to confirm the diagnosis of PD and BPH but especially to distinguish PD individuals from those with MSA [26]. A retrospective study of 23 men with PD who underwent TURP due to BOO secondary to BPH and followed for 3 years after surgery showed the restoration of voiding in nine patients (64 %), while only five patients (36 %) required catheterization [27]. This study concluded that TURP for BPH in patients with PD may be successful in up to 70 % of patients, and the risk of de novo urinary incontinence is minimal.

Even if there is a lack of long-term and randomized studies performed on large cohorts, data available regarding patients with NB and organic BOO due to BPH suggest that conservative treatment and the use of alpha-blockers in mild/moderate obstruction offers limited but positive voiding improvement with poor results in patients with more severe neurological impairments [28, 29]. When surgery becomes advisable due to medical treatment failure, an adequate history, symptoms assessment, and physical examination potentially supported by sphincter electromyography (EMG) and urodynamic or videourodynamic studies can help to identify those individuals with high risk of postoperative urinary incontinence [30].

12.3   Surgical Treatment BOO in NB Women

There are no specific studies performed on large cohorts and with long-term follow-up regarding the management of BOO secondary to pelvic organ prolapse (POP) in women suffering from NB. Ruffion et al. in 2007 emphasized the particular risks of the surgical approaches in these patients in view of the limited literature on the subject [31]. Therefore, indications for POP surgery remain those for general population, but a very careful preoperative evaluation is mandatory. In fact POP symptoms can be often mystifying, and it may be difficult to correlate specific symptoms with the site or severity of POP [32]. This statement should be taken into strong consideration especially in NB women considering that more than two thirds of parous women have objective evidence of POP at clinical examination and that the majority of these defects are asymptomatic and fewer than 15 % of them will require surgical intervention [33]. However, when complications become recurrent, QoL and sexual function are hardly compromised, and when conservative treatments (including devices as pessaries) fail, surgery should be indicated. Otherwise from uncomplicated SUI or prolapsed where routine preoperative urodynamic evaluation is still controversial, urodynamic or videourodynamic with striated sphincter electromyography are strongly recommended in patients with NB and POP. This with the aim to comprehensively evaluate and categorize the associated bladder dysfunction (detrusor overactivity, possible occult stress urinary incontinence, underactive bladder) allowing the clinician to predict the final outcome of the surgical treatment and inform patients about potential postoperative consequences and relative therapeutic options available.

12.4   Final Considerations

Surgery management of BOO in NB either in males and in females may represent a challenge and a specialized management is required. Surgery becomes mandatory in case of severe and recurrent complications or when QoL is so compromised to require a surgical intervention. Patients have to be accurately evaluated by urological and neurophysiological examinations with the aim to assess the risk of postoperative consequences and properly inform patients. In fact, depending on type of NB dysfunction, after BOO surgery, some symptoms may improve but some others may worsen. Therefore, patients should preoperatively know which could be the possible postoperative residual symptoms and which possible subsequent therapeutic options will be available. Patients with detrusor overactivity might develop or worsen urge urinary incontinence, while those suffering from underactive bladder should need self-bladder catheterization despite surgical treatment. As a final consideration, beyond the medical goals, treatment choice has to be definitely shared with our patients in order to customize, whenever possible, the therapeutic algorithm basing not only on clinical indications but also on patients personality, lifestyles, and expectations. Furthermore, after surgery has been performed, a rigorous follow-up is recommended to check that the therapeutic effects are maintained during the time and to prevent the onset of long-term complications or BOO recurrence.

References

1. Paul Abrams, Linda Cardozo, Saad Khoury, Alan Wein. Incontinence.
2. European Association of Urology Guidelines.
3. Abrams P, Cardozo L, Fall M, Griffiths D, Rosier P, Ulmstein U. The standardization of terminology of lower urinary tract function. Report from the standardization committee of the international continence society. Neurourol Urodyn. 2002;21(7):167–78.
4. Block BF. Central pathways controlling micturition and urinary incontinence. Urology. 2002;59(5):13–7.
5. Utomo E, Groen J, Blok BFM. Surgical management of functional bladder outlet obstruction in adults with neurogenic bladder dysfunction (review). Cochrane Database Syst Rev. 2014;5:CD004927.
6. Pan D, Troy A, Rogerson J, Bolton D, Brown D, Lawrentschuk N. Long term outcomes of external sphincterotomy in a spinal injure population. J Urol. 2009;181(2):705–9.
7. Shaw PJ, Milroy E, Timoney AG, el Din A, Mitchell N. Permanent external striated sphincter stents in patients with spinal injuries. Br J Urol. 1990;66(3):292–302.
8. Chancellor MB, Gajewski J, Ackman CF, Appell RA, Bennett J, Binard J, et al. Long term follow-up of the North American Multicenter UroLume trial for the treatment of external detrusor sphincter dyssynergia. J Urol. 1999;161(5):1545–50.
9. Chancellor MB, Hirsch IH, Kiilholma P, Staas WE. Technique of external sphincter balloon dilatation. Urology. 1992;40(4):308–10.
10. Chancellor MB, Rivas DA, Abdil CK, Karasick S, Ehrlich SM, Staas WE. Prospective comparison of external urethral sphincter dilatation and prosthesis placement with external sphincterotomy in spinal cord injured men. Arch Phys Med Rehabil. 1994;75(3):297–305.
11. Mc Farlane JP, Foley SJ, Shah PJ. Balloon dilatation of the external urethral sphincter in the treatment of detrusor sphincter dyssynergia. Spinal Cord. 1997;3582:96–8.
12. Dykstra DD, Sidi AA, Scott AB, Pagel JM, Goldfish GD. Effects of botulinum A toxin on detruso-sphincter dyssynergia in spinal cord injury patients. J Urol. 1988;139(5):919–22.
13. Schurch B, Hauri D, Rodic B, Curt A, Meyer M, Rossier AB. Botulinum-A toxin as treatment of detrusor sphincter dyssynergia: a prospective study in 24 spinal cord injury patients. J Urol. 1996;155(3):1023–9.
14. Steers WD, Meythaler JM, Haworth C, Herrell D, Parks TS. Effects of acute bolus and chronic continuous intrathecal baclofen on genitourinary dysfunction due to spinal cord pathology. J Urol. 1992;148(6):1849–55.
15. Myazzato M, Sasatomi K, Hiragata S, Sugaya K, Chancellor MB, de Groat WC. Suppression of detrusor sphincter dyssynergia by GABA-receptor activation in the lumbosacral spinal cord in spinal cord injured rats. Am J Physiol Regul Integr Comp Physiol. 2008;295(1):R336–42.
16. Ko HY, Kim KT. Treatment of external urethral sphincter hypertonicity by pudendal nerve blocking using phenol solution in patients with spinal cord injury. Spinal Cord. 1997;35(10):690–3.

17. Tsai SJ, Lew HL, Date E, Bih LI. Treatment of detrusor-sphincter dyssynergia by pudendal nerve block in patients with spinal cord injury. Arch Phys Med Rehabil. 2002;83(5):714–7.
18. Koyanagi T, Morita H, Takamatsu T, Taniguchi K, Shinno Y. Radical transurethral resection of the prostate in male paraplegics revisited: further clinical experience and urodynamic considerations for its effectiveness. J Urol. 1987;137(1):72–6.
19. Sakakibara R, Panicker J, Finazzi agro E, Iacovelli V, Bruschini H, The Parkinson's Disease Sub-Committee. The neurourology promotion committee in the international continence society. Neurourol Urodyn. 2015;25:1–13.
20. Goldstein DS, Sewell L, Sharabi Y. Autonomic dysfunction in PD: a window to early detection? J Neurol Sci. 2011;310(1-2):118–22.
21. Soler JM, Le Portz B. Bladder sphincter disorders in Parkinson's disease. Ann Urol. 2004;38:S57–61.
22. Stocchi F, Carbone A, Inghilleri M, Frongillo D, Barbato L, Bramante L, Cannata D, Manfredi M, Ruggieri S. Instrumental diagnosis of multiple system atrophy. Adv Neurol. 1996;69:421–4.
23. Stocchi F, Carbone A, Inghilleri M, Monge A, Ruggieri S, Manfredi M. J Neurol Neurosurg Psychiatry. 1997;62(5):507–11.
24. Fowler CJ. Update on the neurology of Parkinson's disease. Neurourol Urodyn. 2007;26:103–9.
25. Perez-Lloret S, Rey MV, Pavy-Le Traon A, et al. Emerging drugs for autonomic dysfunction in Parkinson's disease. Expert Opin Emerg Drugs. 2013;18:39–53.
26. Fowler CJ, Dalton C, Panicker JN. Review of neurologic diseases for the urologist. Urol Clin N Am. 2010;37:517–26; Defreitas GA, Lemack GE, Zimmern PE, et al. Distinguishing neurogenic from non-neurogenic detrusor overactivity: a urodynamic assessment of lower urinary tract symptoms in patients with and without Parkinsons disease. Urology. 2003;62:651–5.
27. Roth B, Studer UE, Fowler CJ, et al. Benign prostatic obstruction and Parkinson's disease should transurethral resection of the prostate be avoided. J Urol. 2009;181:2209–13.
28. Ransmayr GN, Holliger S, Schletterer K, et al. Lower urinary tract symptoms in dementia with Lewy bodies, Parkinson disease, and Alzheimer disease. Neurology. 2008;70:299–303.
29. Gomes CM, Sammour ZM, Bessa Jr J, et al. Predicting response to doxazosin in patients with voiding dysfunction and Parkinson disease: impact of the neurological impairment. Neurourol Urodyn. 2010;29:313.
30. Winge K, Fowler CJ. Bladder dysfunction in Parkinsonism: mechanisms, prevalence, symptoms, and management. Mov Disord. 2006;21:737–45.
31. Ruffion A, Chartier-Kastler E. Specific features of genital prolapse in spinal cord injury patients. Prog Urol. 2007;17(3):440–1.
32. Swift SE, Tate SB, Nicholas J. Correlation of symptoms with degree of pelvic organ support in a general population of women: what is pelvic organ prolapse? Am J Obstet Gynecol. 2003;189(2):372–7; discussion 377–9.
33. Bump RC, Norton PA. Epidemiology and natural history of pelvic floor dysfunction. Obstet Gynecol Clin N Am. 1998;25:723–46.

Botulinum Toxin Bladder Injection in the Treatment of Neurogenic Detrusor Overactivity and Idiopathic OAB

13

Vincenzo Li Marzi, Jacopo Frizzi, Matteo Bonifazi, and Giulio Del Popolo

13.1   Introduction

Over the last 50 years, botulinum toxin (BoNT) has been transformed from a cause of life-threatening disease to an effective therapy, mainly for muscle spasticity, blepharospasm, and bladder overactivity. It has been used for different indications in a variety of medical specialties as treatment, improving patient's quality of life [1]. There are eight types of BoNT, named from A to H, and BoNT/A type represents the most used for human therapy. A recent growing body of evidence suggests that intradetrusor injection of BoNT/A may have beneficial effects in patients with refractory detrusor overactivity (DO) for conservative and/or medical treatments, and it is a new minimally invasive alternative to bladder augmentation in patients with severe overactive bladder (OAB) symptoms and/or untreatable neurogenic bladder.

Urinary urgency (UU), urge incontinence (UI), urinary frequency (UF), and nocturia are symptoms that characterize the OAB syndrome. In patients with only UU and UF, OAB is defined as "dry"; meanwhile it is defined "wet" if it is associated with UI.

The physiological basis of these symptoms is DO, defined as an involuntary detrusor contraction during the filling phase of urodynamic studies. DO may be spontaneous or provoked and may also be qualified according to cause in neurogenic or idiopathic [2].

V. Li Marzi (✉) • J. Frizzi • M. Bonifazi
Department of Urology, Careggi University Hospital, Florence, Italy
e-mail: vlimarzi@hotmail.com

G. Del Popolo
Neurourology Unit, Careggi University Hospital, Florence, Italy

© Springer International Publishing Switzerland 2016
A. Carbone et al. (eds.), *Functional Urologic Surgery in Neurogenic and Oncologic Diseases*, Urodynamics, Neurourology and Pelvic Floor Dysfunctions, DOI 10.1007/978-3-319-29191-8_13

Urodynamic diagnosis of neurogenic detrusor overactivity (NDO) is always associated with a documented neurologic diseases. On the other hand, DO that is not clearly associated with neurologic cause or with a clearly obvious other cause (e.g., bladder stone, bladder cancer, UTI) has an urodynamic diagnosis of idiopathic detrusor overactivity (IDO) [2].

The use of intradetrusor BoNT for the treatment of DO has revolutionized the care of patients with OAB [3].

13.2 What Is NDO?

The normal function of the lower urinary tract in storage and voiding of urine is coordinated by neural control within the brain and spinal cord. Consequently, any interruption to this system affecting bladder or outflow function may lead to symptoms of neurogenic bladder or neurogenic lower urinary tract dysfunction (NLUTD). Patients with NLUTD usually are symptomatic and may be at risk of long-term complications, the most significant of which is damage of renal function. This is secondary to high bladder storage pressures with or without vesico-ureteral reflux [4]. Elevated bladder pressure is due to detrusor overactivity and/or poor bladder compliance during storage, as well as detrusor muscle contractions against a closed sphincter known as detrusor sphincter dyssynergia. The nature and extent of symptoms is dependent on the type of pathology, severity, and location within the nervous system. Therefore, treatment and long-term management varies according to the underlying disease process and resulting symptoms [5].

The relative risk of developing NLUTD in relation to specific pathologies is better understood. It often accompanies spinal cord injury, basal ganglia diseases, demyelinating disorders, and cerebrovascular diseases. The causes of spinal cord injury are multifactorial. They can be traumatic, vascular, congenital, or medical in origin. Patients with lesions above T10 with upper motor neuron-type injury will suffer from NLUTD consisting of neurogenic detrusor overactivity and detrusor sphincter dyssynergia. Those with lesions below L2 and a lower motor neuron-type injury will likely have an acontractile detrusor [6]. Many patients develop NDO as a result of neurologic conditions such as multiple sclerosis (MS) or spinal cord injury (SCI). NDO frequently results in urinary incontinence (UI), which has been shown to significantly impair nearly all aspects of patients' health-related quality of life (HRQoL) and may further compound the disability associated with their condition. Life satisfaction has also been shown to be significantly lower among SCI patients with continence problems compared with individuals with bladder control [1]. NDO is defined as detrusor overactivity associated with a neurologic condition, so it is an aspect of NLUTD. NDO occurs when a known neurologic abnormality impairs the signaling systems between the bladder and the central nervous system, and the brain is unable to inhibit the detrusor muscles [6]. NDO is commonly associated with spinal cord injury (SCI) and multiple sclerosis (MS), but patients with cerebrovascular accident, dementia, Parkinson's disease, and other neurologic diseases may develop NDO. Any supra-sacral spinal cord lesions can cause NDO. The majority of people, however, that have been systematically studied are adults with MS and SCI and children and young adults with myelodysplasia [2, 7, 8].

13.3 What Is Idiopathic OAB?

OAB syndrome is defined as urgency, with or without UI, in the absence of pathological or metabolic disorders (bladder outlet obstruction, known neurological conditions, urinary tract infections) that might otherwise cause such symptoms. It is often associated with frequency and nocturia and affects 12–17% of individuals worldwide [1–9]. Approximately one-third of people with OAB have UUI [2]. OAB may negatively impact quality of life, work productivity, mental health, and sleep quality. Additionally, there is increased risk of infections, falls, and fractures particularly in elderly subjects [3].

The underlying pathophysiology associated with idiopathic OAB is widely acknowledged to be multifactorial. Symptoms of urgency, the hallmark feature of idiopathic OAB, are thought to result from increased activity or hypersensitivity afferents in the urothelial mucosal layer of the bladder, or overactivity of the detrusor muscle, or abnormal central nervous system processing of bladder afferent signaling [10, 11].

Urothelial or suburothelial dysfunction has been hypothesized to elicit OAB symptoms due to changes in the bladder mucosa at the level of the stratified urothelium or the interstitial cells of the lamina propria [12, 13]. The urothelium is also a sensory tissue expressing a wide range of signaling molecules and membrane receptors and responds to mechanical and chemical stimulation that may contribute to bladder sensation which could be altered for an increased afferent nerve expression [12–14]. Interstitial cells may play a role in the development of idiopathic OAB with modified expression of various interstitial cell markers (e.g., gap junction proteins). These kinds of proteins are expressed in toxic or inflammatory-mediated signaling, increasing the activation of suburothelial sensory afferents [12–15].

The myogenic hypothesis of OAB suggested that derived symptoms of OAB originate from upregulated, spontaneous, or involuntary contractions of detrusor muscle cells [15].

Abnormal central processing of bladder afferent signaling and/or cognitive manipulation has been proposed to produce perceptions of UU in idiopathic OAB patients [10].

Elements that could contribute to the "brain factor," as a supposed mechanism for eliciting sensations of UU, include alterations in the normal regulation by the insula, prefrontal cortex, and anterior cingulate gyrus, as well as the presence of environmental triggers or some effective states or psychological factors like anxiety that induce the expression of stress-related peptides which exacerbate chronic syndromes such as interstitial cystitis and OAB [16].

13.4   What Is the Treatment for NDO and Idiopathic OAB?

European Association of Urology (EAU) guidelines recommended as first-line treatment for OAB behavior modifications or simply educating patients to be more strategic with regard to their fluid intake habits and other lifestyle factors that may be associated with incontinence, including obesity, smoking, level of physical activity, and diet [17].

The fact that urinary symptoms were demonstrated to be exacerbated by excessive caffeine intake has focused attention on whether reduced consumption of coffee or drinks containing caffeine such as tea and cola may improve UI [17, 18]. Modifications in fluid intake, particularly restriction, are a strategy commonly used by people with UI to relieve symptoms. A recent RCT showed that a reduction in fluid intake by 25 % improved symptoms in patients with OAB but not UI [19].

Obesity has been identified as a risk factor for UI in many epidemiological studies. There is evidence that the prevalence of both UUI and stress urinary incontinence (SUI) increases proportionately with rising body mass index. Smoking, especially if more than 20 cigarettes per day, is considered to intensify UI [18]. Identifying exacerbating factors, modifying behavior patterns, reducing infections, biofeedback, and pelvic floor strengthening are the mainstay of conservative management.

American Urological Association (AUA) guidelines published in 2014 on the management of OAB confirm the role of behavioral therapy as first-line approach and pharmacologic therapy as second-line approach [20]. Antimuscarinic therapy is the mainstay of medical therapy for OAB. However, compliance has been poor, and discontinuation rates have been high due to the lack of efficacy and adverse side effects [20, 21]. The beta-agonist mirabegron has recently been approved for the management of OAB; however, its impact on patient's compliance is yet to be determined in the long-term follow-up. Mirabegron is the first clinically available beta-3 agonist, and it reduces the incontinence episodes, urgency episodes, and micturition frequency/24 h. Beta-3 adrenoreceptors are the predominant beta receptors expressed in smooth muscle cells of the detrusor, and their stimulation is thought to induce detrusor relaxation [21].

Also in patients with NDO, antimuscarinic drugs represent the first-line choice. More recently, mirabegron was employed in some clinical experiences, but studies on safety and effectiveness in NDO patients are ongoing [17].

The third-line OAB treatment, only in idiopathic patients, has relied on sacral neuromodulation, such as sacral nerve stimulation, which requires minimally invasive surgical intervention [20]. Sacral neuromodulation is associated with a surgical revision rate of 3–16 % and was first approved for IDO in urological field [22]. Peripheral tibial nerve stimulation (PTNS) may be offered as the third-line treatment in a carefully selected idiopathic patient population [20].

Intradetrusor injection of onabotulinumtoxinA was approved in 2011 for the management of NDO. In January 2013, it was approved for the management of "wet OAB" [20–23]. In this type of third-line treatment, associated intermittent catheterization must be taken in consideration.

In selected patients, augmentation cystoplasty or urinary diversion for severe, refractory, complicated OAB patients may be considered, especially in subjects with very small anatomical bladder [20–23].

13.5 History of Botulinum Toxin in Urology: Development and Mechanism of Action

The BoNT is a neurotoxic protein causing a severe flaccid paralysis and synthesized by *Clostridium botulinum*, a Gram-positive obligated anaerobe bacterium.

The first incident of food-borne botulism was documented in the eighteenth century, when the consumption of meat and blood sausages gave rise to many deaths throughout the kingdom of Württemberg, in southwestern Germany. The district medical officer, Justinus Kerner (1786–1862), who was also a well-known German poet, published the first accurate and complete descriptions of the symptoms of food-borne botulism between 1817 and 1822 and attributed the intoxication to a biological poison. In 1895, an outbreak of botulism in the small Belgian village of Ellezelles led to the discovery of the pathogen *Clostridium botulinum* by Emile Pierre van Ermengem. Modern botulinum toxin treatment was pioneered by Alan B. Scott and Edward J. Schantz in the early 1970s, when type A serotype was used in medicine to correct strabismus [24].

Actually eight serotypes of BoNT are described, and only types A, B, E, F, and H cause human disease. They are resistant to degradation by enzymes of gastrointestinal tract, and they are absorbed from the intestinal mucosa into the bloodstream [25].

The BoNT is a two-chain protein composed of heavy chain polypeptides joined via disulfide bonds to light chain polypeptides. The eight serologically distinct toxin types possess different tertiary structures and significant sequence divergences.

The molecular target of the toxin type A (BoNT/A) is the synaptosomal-associated protein 25 (SNAP-25), a protein involved in vesicle fusion and mediating release of acetylcholine, from axon endings. A new hypothesis of afferent BoNT/A mechanism of action in the bladder combines the presynaptic cholinergic junction inducing detrusor muscle relaxation to an action on afferent sensory receptors in the urothelium. Emerging data suggest that these sensory effects are probably due to the action of BoNT/A on neurotransmitters other than acetylcholine. The BoNT/A seems to have an antinociceptive action, independent of its neuromuscular junction-blocking action, that might involve modulation of glutamate, substance P, calcitonin gene-related peptide, enkephalins, and others [5, 26].

BoNT/A was first approved in humans as medical therapy for the treatment of benign essential blepharospasm and strabismus in 1989 with the TM Botox®. The use of BoNT/A in the urinary tract was first describe by Dykstra et al. in 1988, who injected it into the external urinary sphincter to treat detrusor sphincter dyssynergia in patients with spinal cord injury [27]. Its use is expanded in the management of lower urinary tract symptoms associated with detrusor overactivity, bladder outflow obstruction, and painful bladder syndrome/interstitial cystitis. BoNT/A is most commonly used in the management of lower urinary tract symptoms. Occasionally, BoNT/B has been used in few patients resistant to previous BoNT/A treatment [28, 29].

Currently, there are three commonly used formulations of BoNT/A: *onabotulinumtoxinA* (Botox or Vistabel – Allergen, Irvine, CA, USA), *abobotulinumtoxinA* (Dysport – Medicis, Scottsdale, AZ, USA, or Azzalure – Ipsen, Paris, France), and *incobotulinumtoxinA* (Xeomin or Bocouture – Merz Pharmaceuticals, Frankfurt, Germany). This accounts for the variations in dose, efficacy, duration of effect, and safety profile of the different preparations. Largest series and approval studies in urological field are regarding onabotulinumtoxinA.

13.6 Bladder Injection Technique

The target layer within the bladder wall for cystoscopic intravesical injection is generally considered to be the detrusor muscle. Cystoscopic visualization is not accurate in assessing the depth of needle penetration into the bladder wall. A submucosal blush "bleb" implies the needle is submucosal. A slight bulge at site of injection implies muscle is probably included [30, 31].

The absence of visual dye changes at the site of injection may suggest that the needle tip is at serosal or extravesical level. Another variable that may influence which layer of the bladder wall is injected (apart from the length/depth of the injecting needle) is bladder wall thickness which depends on patient age, the presence of bladder outflow obstruction, and the degree of fullness of the bladder [32, 33].

Kuo assesses that BoNT/A suburothelial injections are more effective than detrusor injections in IDO patients to reduce significant voiding difficulty, but nevertheless, 30 % required catheterization [34]. The author proposes that the blockage of detrusor muscle through suburothelial sensory fibers was more pronounced than neuromuscular junctions and/or the small amount of BoNT/A diffusion from the detrusor to the suburothelium – following detrusor injection – was responsible for the responses previously reported [34].

A recent study examines the later distribution of BoNT/A/gadolinium within the bladder wall by performing a delayed MRI scan at 3 h after intravesical injection, trying to explain how BoNT/A may be producing its effect. Twenty consecutive patients were enrolled (8 males, 12 females): 9 have IDO and 11 have NDO. Fourteen patients repeated the procedures, and six received intravesical BoNT/A injection for the first time. Patients received a total of 20 injections of 1 ml into bladder wall sites, including 2 injections into the trigone. According to this study, the diffusion of BoNT/A after intravesical injection appears to be very common once the mucosa and the detrusor muscle are pricked. Therefore, precise injection localization, specifically into the detrusor muscle layer at cystoscopy, may not be as relevant to the outcome as previously assumed [35]. Another paper confirms that BoNT/A injections in the bladder wall can spread the toxin to areas very distant from the injection point [36].

Currently approved procedure expected that the bladder should be filled gradually to ensure adequate visualization, but it should not be overdistended. Intradetrusor injections of 100 U and 200 U of onabotulinumtoxinA are dosages approved for "wet"

OAB and NDO, respectively. Dilution in 20 ml of saline solution for "wet" OAB and 30 ml for NDO is recommended. The intradetrusor injections are performed by means of cystoscopy at 1 cm distance from each other, sparing the trigone, for a total of 20 injections in iOAB "wet" patients, and 30 injections in the NDO patients.

The depth of the injection is fundamental to avoid systemic side effects. It is recommended that the injection should be approximately 2 mm into the detrusor. If the injection is too superficial, a mound would be created. Theoretically, if the injection is too superficial, the onabotulinumtoxinA could leak through the puncture site or will not diffuse into the detrusor muscle. If the injection is placed too deep, the toxin may diffuse into the surrounding structures [37, 38].

The use of suburothelial injection compared to intradetrusor injection was evaluated in a study of 32 patients with neurogenic bladder secondary to SCI. The only parameter favoring intradetrusor injection was the improvement in detrusor compliance. No other differences in the short-term follow-up between intradetrusor and suburothelial injections were noted for number of catheterizations in 24 h, number of incontinence episodes in 24 h, catheterized volume, cystometric bladder capacity, volume at first involuntary detrusor contraction, and maximum detrusor pressure during filling [39].

Needles for intradetrusor injection of onabotulinumtoxinA vary in size from 20 to 25 gauge. The tip length varies from 2.5 to 8 mm, and the overall length of the injection needle varies from 31.3 to 105 cm. It is important for clinicians to be aware of the differences between needles because these differences may affect injection technique and patient comfort. Significant bleeding is rarely encountered during the injection, but patients should be informed that blood in the urine may occur for a day or two after the procedure. When performing the injections with the use of a flexible cystoscope, it is important to either use a needle with an introducer tip or pre-place the needle with its tip just inside the working channel prior to passing the scope into the bladder. Failure to do so may cause damage to the working channel.

Prophylactic antibiotic therapy is recommended [38–41]. The use of indwelling catheter is not mandatory but depends on clinician judgment. Upon completion of the procedure, patients who are not on clean intermittent catheterization should be observed to ensure they are able to void prior to discharge, and post-void residual should be measured. The onset of action can take 1–2 weeks. Post-void residual should be remeasured approximately 2 weeks post-procedure. The choice to start clean intermittent catheterization is based on the post-void residual volume and presence of symptoms. Efficacy is typically observed 6–9 months postinjection [41]. Patients should not be retreated prior to 12 weeks postinjection.

13.7 Botulinum Toxin A for NDO and Idiopathic "Wet" OAB

13.7.1 Efficacy in NDO

There is an established evidence-based and reported high level of evidence (LE) data for the use of onabotulinumtoxinA (Botox) in the treatment of NDO and idiopathic "wet" OAB (wet iOAB) and abobotulinumtoxinA (Dysport) for NDO only [8]. BoNT/A causes a long-lasting but reversible chemical denervation that lasts for about 9 months in neuro-urological patients. The toxin injections are mapped over the detrusor in a dosage that depends on the preparation used [8]. In NDO patients, three studies were LE1, two onabotulinumtoxinA and one abobotulinumtoxinA [8].

Ehren et al. have compared abobotulinumtoxinA 500 units with placebo and found it to significantly reduce the need for anticholinergic medication [42]. Del Popolo et al. study using this preparation randomized patients to either 500 or 750 units. The authors found a trend toward greater improvement with 750 units that was not significant [21].

OnabotulinumtoxinA has been proven effective in patients with neuro-urological disorders in phase III RCTs [43]. In phase III RCTs, onabotulinumtoxinA 200 and 300 units has been shown to lead to significant improvements in parameters compared to placebo [5, 43–45]. Moreover, no significant differences were found between 200 and 300 U dosage for efficacy and duration, so 200 U is the approved dosage in NDO patients. Although one study reported a slightly higher rate of completely "dry" patients receiving 300 units (41 %) compared to 200 units of onabotulinumtoxinA (36 %) at 6 weeks posttreatment [46].

A systematic review (28 studies included) of the efficacy and safety of botulinum toxin A intradetrusor injections in adults with NDO demonstrated superior effects of onabotulinumtoxinA compared with placebo in continence, reduction in incontinence episodes, improvement in urodynamic parameters, as well as improvement in health-related quality-of-life assessments. The most commonly encountered side effects were the need for clean intermittent catheterization, urinary retention, and urinary tract infections. In this review, the dose of onabotulinumtoxinA used for NDO ranged from 100 to 300 units [47]. Schurch et al. also noted a difference in the continence status between patients treated with 200 units of onabotulinumtoxinA (23.77 %) compared to placebo (8.5 %) [48]. All studies reported significant reductions in the number of incontinence episodes with both 200 and 300 units of onabotulinumtoxinA [47]. Ginsberg et al. noted that 36 % of patients ($n=135$) treated with 200 units of onabotulinumtoxinA were continent compared to 10 % with placebo ($n=149$) at 6 weeks posttreatment, which was statistically significant [46].

A long-term study by Kennelly et al. demonstrated a sustained, clinically meaningful improvement in urinary symptoms and QOL following onabotulinumtoxinA treatment in patients with UI due to NDO during the 4-year study, with no new safety signals [49]. These results further support the use of onabotulinumtoxinA 200 units in patients with NDO and UI who are inadequately managed by anticholinergic medication. Of the 691 patients enrolled in the phase III study, 396 MS and SCI patients entered the extension study. Data for patients who received at least up to six sequential onabotulinumtoxinA treatments are reported. Patients who needed seven or more treatments during the 4-year study were not large and only one patient received 13 treatments. At week 6 following each treatment, onabotulinumtoxinA 200 units consistently reduced the mean number of daily UI episodes. The proportion of patients achieving 50 % reduction in UI episodes/day was consistently over

83%, whereas the percent of patients with a 100% reduction in UI episodes/day ranged from 43% to 56% across six treatments. Repeated injections were demonstrated to be possible without loss of efficacy [49].

13.7.2 Efficacy iOAB Wet

An approval study with a phase III placebo-controlled trial of onabotulinumtoxinA in 557 patients with wet iOAB inadequately managed with anticholinergics was performed to obtain approval for this kind of treatment. At baseline, patients experienced a mean of 5.3 UI episodes per day, most of which were UUI episodes (mean of 4.6 episodes per day). At week 12, there was a mean 47.9% reduction from baseline for onabotulinumtoxinA group vs. 12.5% for placebo. Further, 57.5% of patients treated with onabotulinumtoxinA achieved a 50% or greater reduction in UI episodes compared to 28.9% with placebo. Continence (100% reduction) was achieved by 22.9% of patients treated with onabotulinumtoxinA compared to 6.5% of those receiving placebo [41]. Secondary endpoints included decrease from baseline at week 12 in mean micturition, urgency, and nocturia, as well as impact on patient health-related quality of life using the Incontinence Quality of Life (I-QOL) and Kings Health Questionnaire (KHQ). Statistically significant differences between onabotulinumtoxinA and placebo were noted for all of these secondary endpoints [41].

In another randomized, double-blind, placebo-controlled trial published few months later compared to the Nitti's publication, onabotulinumtoxinA significantly decreased UI episodes per day at week 12 (−2.95 for onabotulinumtoxinA vs. −1.03 for placebo; $p < 0.001$). Reductions from baseline in all other OAB symptoms were also significantly greater following onabotulinumtoxinA compared with placebo ($p \leq 0.01$) [23].

13.7.3 Adverse Events

There are two categories of treatment-related adverse events (AEs) secondary to intradetrusor injection of BoNT/A: local and systemic side effects.

The most common local events are infections and hematuria, which are often related to the procedure rather than to the toxin [5].

The rate of UTI is reported at 21%–32% and injection-associated pain at 10%. These local AEs are more common in patients with IDO than the ones with NDO. In fact, in patients with IDO, the most frequently reported AE is UTI, most cases of which occurred in the first 12 weeks (43 of 278 or 15.5% for onabotulinumtoxinA vs. 16 of 272 or 5.9% for placebo) [44].

Other AEs that occurred in the first 12 weeks at a higher incidence in patients treated with onabotulinumtoxinA are dysuria (12.2%) and bacteriuria (5.0%) [41]. Rarely there are complicated UTIs with upper urinary tract involvement as pyelonephritis [45].

Intradetrusor injections of BoNT/A could be associated with excess weakness or relaxation of the muscles resulting in an underactive detrusor activity with temporary increased risk of post-void residual volume or urinary retention that is a problem for non-neurological patient, and therefore they need to be willing and able to perform intermittent catheterization (IC) if not already doing so [41], meanwhile complete urinary retention is what we try to obtain in patient with NDO that are used to perform IC.

Nitti et al. describe a PVR significantly increased in patients with IDO treated with onabotulinumtoxinA vs. placebo with the highest volume at posttreatment week 2. At weeks 2, 6, and 12, values were 49.5, 42.1, and 32.6 ml in the onabotulinumtoxinA group vs. 1.1, 3.1, and 2.5 ml in the placebo group, respectively. Of the 276 patients, 24 (8.7%) exhibited a 200 ml or great increase from baseline in PVR at any time after initial treatment with onabotulinumtoxinA vs. none treated with placebo. The proportion of patients who initiated IC at any time during treatment cycle 1 was 6.1% (17/278) vs. none in the placebo group. For more than half the patients who initiated IC (10/17), the duration was 6 weeks or less [41].

Chapple et al. in their study report that the majority of patients with IDO (75.8%) did not have an increase from baseline in PVR >100 ml following treatment with onabotulinumtoxinA 100 U, and only 8.8% of patients in the onabotulinumtoxinA group had a change from baseline in PVR 200 ml at any point during the treatment cycle. The proportion of patients who initiated IC following onabotulinumtoxinA treatment was 6.9%. IC was started in nearly all patients within the first 12 weeks following treatment; only two patients in the placebo group (0.7%) initiated IC [45].

Urinary retention could be a dose-related side effect, for example, Rajkumar et al. report an increased post-void residual volume in some patients with IDO after 300 UI BoNT/A [50]. Kuo et al. describe an increased dose-related risk of urinary retention and bad bladder emptying (100 U: 0%; 150 U: 10%; 200 U: 20%) [31].

In neurological non-catheterizing patients, Cruz et al. have demonstrated an augmented incidence of de novo IC with the increase of the dosage, respectively, 12% for placebo, 30% 200 U, and 42% 300 U. In addition, patients submitted to reinjection reported a lower incidence of urinary retention [43].

Systemic events occur due to migration of toxin beyond the detrusor muscle causing muscle weakness or hyposthenia in nontargeted adjacent muscles or distal ones. The incidence of severe adverse events as diaphragmatic paralysis is very low. General hyposthenia was first reported in 2001 during the 18th International Continence Society Meeting [51]. The incidence of severe adverse events in high-level studies in patients receiving BoNT/A is low. It must be noted that the majority of cases of hyposthenia are transient and mild [52].

Del Popolo et al. report hyposthenia and muscle weakness in 5 of 61 patients (8%) treated with 1000 U of abobotulinumtoxinA for NDO [53]. These effects persist for about 4 weeks after injection. Furthermore, Grosse et al. describe that four patients (17%) had transient muscle weakness in the trunk and/or extremities lasting up to 2 months [54].

Controlled clinical trials are needed to establish the optimum dose and technical details of administering BoNT/A, the number of injection sites, the volume of dilution, and whether the trigone should be spared, as these have not yet been specifically determined and can play an important role to maximize efficacy and avoid side effects. It's important to underline that none of the major BoNT/A-related side effects are observed with approved therapeutic dosages.

13.8 Future Research

A promising role in the treatment of NDO and iOAB is represented by the use of intravesical injections of liposomes, either empty or filled with specific drugs.

Liposomes are lipid vesicles composed of concentric phospholipid bilayers enclosing an aqueous interior [55, 56] and have been studied as drug carriers since their capacity of improving the delivery of chemotherapeutic agents while reducing the risk of adverse side effects [57–59].

Empty liposomes have itself a topical healing effect, as seen in ophthalmological conditions such as keratitis, uveitis, endophthalmitis, proliferative vitreoretinopathy, and corneal transplant rejection [60].

For this reason, empty liposomes may be used as therapeutic agents for bladder injury.

Preclinical studies have shown using a rat model of bladder injury, induced by protamine sulfate, that instillation of liposomes protected bladder from irritation [61].

Furthermore, empty liposome instillation has been used as control against capsaicin delivery study, and bladder tolerance was investigated by cystometry and histology [62].

Cystometric studies involved bladder injury induced by protamine sulfate for an hour followed by irritation caused by infusion of high concentration of potassium chloride solution [63, 64]. Posttreatment of liposomes showed the protective effect in this model [63, 64], which involved coadministration of liposomes with potassium chloride to mimic the clinical disease condition. The comparative efficacy of liposomes was evaluated against FDA-approved therapies of dimethyl sulfoxide (DMSO) and intravesical instillation of PPS [65].

Clinically, DMSO (RIMSO-50) is the only FDA-approved intravesical treatment for PBS/IC, [66] but off-label instillation of PPS has also been pursued [67]. The efficacy of various treatments was evaluated in chemically induced bladder hyperactivity in rats by sequential infusion of protamine sulfate and potassium chloride. Bladder reflex activity of female Sprague-Dawley rats before and after treatment was evaluated by continuous cystometry under urethane anesthesia (1.0 g/kg). Intravesical liposomes were effective in doubling the intercontractile interval (ICI) compared with PPS, while acute instillation of DMSO failed to produce any protective effect in this animal model [68]. Encouraged by the exciting preclinical efficacy liposomes as therapeutic agent for intravesical therapy of IC/PBS, Chuang et al. recently published the clinical safety and efficacy of liposomes in IC/PBS patients [69]. In an open-label prospective study on 24 IC/PBS patients, the effect of intravesical liposomes was compared against oral PPS. Patients were equally divided into the two treatment arms, administered either intravesical liposomes (80 mg/40 cc distilled water) once weekly or oral PPS (100 mg) three times daily for 4 weeks each. Ten possible responses to treatment were monitored at three time points, including baseline, and at weeks 4 and 8. Comparable efficacy of liposomes to oral PPS was demonstrated by statistically significant decreases in urinary frequency and nocturia in both treatment arms. Liposome treated patients showed statistically significant decreases in pain, urgency, and the O'Leary-Sant symptom score, with the effect being most profound on urgency. None of the treated patients in the study reported urinary incontinence, retention, or infection due to liposome instillation, and there were no unanticipated adverse events and no significant worsening of symptoms during follow-up. The exact mechanism of action for liposomes in IC/PBS remains to be established, but protective coating effect based on preclinical studies cannot be ruled out. In the field of neuro-urology, liposomes may have a major role in improving delivery of neurotoxins into the bladder to achieve a better chemical neuromodulation of afferent neurotransmission since existing approaches of instillation of the drugs are not optimal because of both the vehicle toxicity and degradation by proteases and proteinases in urine, dilution in urine, and poor uptake of the BoNT solution into the urothelium [70, 71]. Moreover, the use of liposomes can enhance efficacy at lower doses [72], protecting the BoNT entrapped inside the liposomes from degradation in urine without compromising its efficacy, as demonstrated by attenuation of acetic acid-induced bladder irritation in rats [73]. Also its transport into the urothelium from liposomes has been confirmed by detection of its effect on SNAP-25 through immunohistochemistry analysis [73]. Liposomes are an attractive drug delivery platform by virtue of their biodegradability, biocompatibility, low toxicity, and simple and mild preparation methods and thus must be considered as a forefront drug delivery system and treatment to improve pharmacotherapy of bladder diseases in the future.

Conclusions

BoNT/A injections into the detrusor have a significant but temporally limited effect in idiopathic and neurogenic DO resistant to antimuscarinic treatment. Furthermore, the establishment of onabotulinumtoxinA as approved treatment in both NDO and wet iOAB will allow more patients to benefit from this treatment.

Little steps toward a better understanding about the efficacy of BoNT/A and how it works have been taken and a growing body of evidence has been published.

What we know about NDO is that BoNT/A has an extraordinary efficacy in patients with spinal cord lesions even after repeated injections.

What we know about IDO and other urologic not-approved indications (e.g., painful bladder, BPO) is that BoNT/A creates an early amelioration of symptoms. What we need to know is the best method of administration and proper dosage to avoid possible early complications such as urinary retention and long-term complications to detrusor voiding function.

Further researches are needed to avoid the improper usage of BoNT/A because poor results or complications may compromise an opportunity for treatment without precedence in the field of functional urology.

References

1. Sussman D, Patel V, Del Popolo G, et al. Treatment satisfaction and improvement in health-related quality of life with onabotulinumtoxinA in patients with urinary incontinence due to neurogenic detrusor overactivity. Neurourol Urodyn. 2013;32(3):242–9.
2. Abrams P, Cardozo L, Fall M, Standardisation Sub-committee of the International Continence Society, et al. The standardisation of terminology of lower urinary tract function: report from the Standardisation Sub-committee of the International Continence Society. Neurourol Urodyn. 2002;2:167–78.
3. Del Popolo G. Botulinum toxin A era: little steps towards a better understanding. Eur Urol. 2008;54(1):25–7.
4. Gerridzen RG, Thijssen AM, Dehoux E. Risk factors for upper tract deterioration in chronic spinal cord injury patients. J Urol. 1992;147(2):416–8.
5. Mangera A, Apostolidis A, Andersson KE, et al. An updated systematic review and statistical comparison of standardised mean outcomes for the use of botulinum toxin in the management of lower urinary tract disorders. Eur Urol. 2014;65(5):981–90.
6. Burns AS, Rivas DA, Ditunno JF. The management of neurogenic bladder and sexual dysfunction after spinal cord injury. Spine (Phila Pa). 1976;26 Suppl 24:S129–36.
7. Fowler C. Systematic review of therapy for neurogenic detrusor overactivity. Can Urol Assoc J. 2011;5(5 Suppl 2):S146–8.
8. Groen J, Pannek J, Castro Diaz D, Del Popolo G, Gross T, Hamid R, Karsenty G, Kessler TM, Schneider M, 't Hoen L, Blok B. Summary of European Association of Urology (EAU) guidelines on neuro-urology. Eur Urol. 2016;69(2):324–33.
9. Haylen BT, de Ridder D, Freeman RM, Swift SE, Berghmans B, Lee J, Monga A, Petri E, Rizk DE, Sand PK, Schaer GN. An International Urogynecological Association (IUGA)/International Continence Society (ICS) joint report on the terminology for female pelvic floor dysfunction. International Urogynecological Association; International Continence Society. Neurourol Urodyn. 2010;29(1):4–20.
10. Roosen A, Chapple CR, Dmochowski RR, et al. A refocus on the bladder as the originator of storage lower urinary tract symptoms: a systematic review of the latest literature. Eur Urol. 2009;56:810–9.
11. Banakhar MA, Al-Shaiji TF, Hassouna MM. Pathophysiology of overactive bladder. Int Urogynecol J. 2012;23:975–82.
12. Sui GP, Wu C, Roosen A, et al. Modulation of bladder myofibroblast activity: implications for bladder function. Am J Physiol Renal Physiol. 2008;295:F688–97.
13. McCloskey KD. Interstitial cells in the urinary bladder–localization and function. Neurourol Urodyn. 2010;29:82–7.
14. de Groat WC. Highlights in basic autonomic neuroscience: contribution of the urothelium to sensory mechanisms in the urinary bladder. Auton Neurosci. 2013;177:67–71.
15. Ikeda Y, Fry C, Hayashi F, et al. Role of gap junctions in spontaneous activity of the rat bladder. Am J Physiol Renal Physiol. 2007;293:F1018–25.
16. De Wachter S, Smith PP, Tannenbaum C, et al. How should bladder sensation be measured? ICI-RS 2011. Neurourol Urodyn. 2012;31:370–4.
17. Lucas MG, et al. EAU guidelines on urinary incontinence. Partial update March 2015 http://uroweb.org/wp-content/uploads/EAU-Guidelines-Urinary-Incontinence-2015.pdf.
18. Hannestad YS, et al. Are smoking and other lifestyle factors associated with female urinary incontinence? The Norwegian EPINCONT Study. BJOG. 2003;110(3):247–54.
19. Hashim H, et al. How should patients with an overactive bladder manipulate their fluid intake? BJU Int. 2008;102(1):62.
20. Gormley AE, Lightner DJ, Burgio KL, et al. Diagnosis and treatment of overactive bladder (Non-Neurogenic) in adults: AUA/SUFU guideline. https://www.auanet.org/common/pdf/education/clinical-guidance/Overactive-Bladder.pdf.
21. Chapple CR, Cardozo L, Nitti VW, et al. Mirabegron in overactive bladder: a review of efficacy, safety, and tolerability. Neurourol Urodyn. 2014;33(1):17–30.

22. Siddiqui NY, Wu JM, Amundsen CL. Efficacy and adverse events of sacral nerve stimulation for overactive bladder: a systematic review. Neurourol Urodyn. 2010;29 Suppl 1:S18–23. doi:10.1002/nau.20786.

23. Chapple C, Sievert KD, MacDiarmid S, et al. OnabotulinumtoxinA 100 U significantly improves all idiopathic overactive bladder symptoms and quality of life in patients with overactive bladder and urinary incontinence: a randomised, double-blind. Placebo-Control Trial Eur Urol. 2013;64:249–56.

24. Erbguth FJ. From poison to remedy: the chequered history of botulinum toxin. J Neural Transm. 2008;115(4):559–65.

25. Brooks GF, Carroll KC, Butel JS, Morse SA, Mietzner TA Chapter 11. Spore-forming Gram-positive bacilli: bacillus and Clostridium species. In: G.F. Brooks, K.C. Carroll, J.S. Butel, S.A. Morse, T.A. Mietzner (Eds.) Jawetz, Melnick, and Adelberg's medical microbiology. 26th ed. McGraw-Hill, New York; 2013.

26. Bing L. Small molecule inhibitors as countermeasures for botulinum neurotoxin intoxication. Molecules. 2011;16(1):202–20.

27. Dykstra DD, Sidi AA, Scott AB, Pagel JM, Goldish GD. Effects of botulinum A toxin on detrusor-sphincter dyssynergia in spinal cord injury patients. J Urol. 1988;139(5):919–22.

28. Pistolesi D, Selli C, Rossi B, Stampacchia G. Botulinum toxin type B for type A resistant bladder spasticity. J Urol. 2004;171(2 Pt 1):802–3.

29. Reitz A, Schurch B. Botulinum toxin type B injection for management of type A resistant neurogenic detrusor overactivity. J Urol. 2004;171(2 Pt 1):804. discussion 804–5.

30. Mehnert U, Boy S, Schmid M, et al. A morphological evaluation of botulinum neurotoxin A injections into the detrusor muscle using magnetic resonance imaging. World J Urol. 2009;27(3):397–403.

31. Kuo HC. Comparison of effectiveness of detrusor suburothelial and bladder base injections of botulinum toxin A for idiopathic detrusor overactivity. J Urol. 2007;178:1359–63.

32. Hakenberg OW, Linne C, Manseck A, Wirth MP. Bladder wall thickness in normal adults and men with mild lower urinary tract symptoms and benign prostatic enlargement. Neurourol Urodyn. 2000;19(5):585–93.

33. Rule AD, St Sauver JL, Jacobson DJ, et al. Three-dimensional ultrasound bladder characteristics and their association with prostate size and lower urinary tract dysfunction among men in the community. Urology. 2009;74(4):908–13.

34. Kuo HC. Clinical effects of suburothelial injection of botulinum A toxin on patients with non-neurogenic detrusor overactivity refractory to anticholinergics. Urology. 2005;66:94–8.

35. Mazen A, Torreggiani W, Sheikh M, et al. Delayed contrast-enhanced MRI to localize Botox after cystoscopic intravesical injection. Int Urol Nephrol. 2015;47:893–8.

36. Coelho A, Cruz F, Cruz CD, Avelino A. Spread of onabotulinumtoxinA after bladder injection. Experimental study using the distribution of cleaved SNAP-25 as the marker of the toxin action. Eur Urol. 2012;61(6):1178–84.

37. Ikeda Y, Zabbarova IV, Birder LA, de Groat WC, McCarthy CJ, Hanna-Mitchell AT, Kanai AJ. Botulinum neurotoxin serotype A suppresses neurotransmitter release from afferent as well as efferent nerves in the urinary bladder. Eur Urol. 2012;62(6):1157–64.

38. Krhut J, Samal V, Nemec D, Zvara P. Intradetrusor versus suburothelial onabotulinumtoxinA injections for neurogenic detrusor overactivity: a pilot study. Spinal Cord. 2012;50(12):904–7.

39. Krhut J, Samal V, Nemec D, Zvara P. Response to 'Onabotulinum toxin injection in neurogenic detrusor overactivity: intradetrusor versus suburothelial'. Spinal Cord. 2013;51(9):726.

40. Shenot PJ, Mark JR. Intradetrusor onabotulinumtoxinA injection: how i do it. Can J Urol. 2013;20(1):6649–55.

41. Nitti A, et al. OnabotulinumtoxinA for the treatment of patients with overactive bladder and urinary incontinence: results of a phase 3, randomized. Placebo Control Trial J Urol. 2013;189:2186–93.

42. Ehren I, Volz D, Farrelly E, et al. Efficacy and impact of botulinum toxin A on quality of life in patients with neurogenic detrusor overactivity: a randomised, placebo-controlled, double-blind study. Scand J Urol Nephrol. 2007;41(4):335–40.

43. Cruz F, Herschorn S, Aliotta P, et al. Efficacy and safety of onabotulinumtoxinA in patients with urinary incontinence due to neurogenic detrusor overactivity: a randomised, double-blind, placebo-controlled trial. Eur Urol. 2011;60(4):742–50.
44. Mangera A, Andersson KE, Apostolidis A, et al. Contemporary management of lower urinary tract disease with botulinum toxin A: a systematic review of botox (onabotulinumtoxinA) and dysport (abobotulinumtoxinA). Eur Urol. 2011;60(4):784–95.
45. Mehta S, Hill D, McIntyre A, et al. Meta-analysis of botulinum toxin A detrusor injections in the treatment of neurogenic detrusor overactivity after spinal cord injury. Arch Phys Med Rehabil. 2013;94(8):1473–81.
46. Ginsberg D, Gousse A, Keppenne V, et al. Phase 3 efficacy and tolerability study of onabotulinumtoxinA for urinary incontinence from neurogenic detrusor overactivity. J Urol. 2012; 187(6):2131–9.
47. Soljanik I. Efficacy and safety of botulinum toxin A intradetrusor injections in adults with neurogenic detrusor overactivity/neurogenic overactive bladder: a systematic review. Drugs. 2013;73(10):1055–66. doi:10.1007/s40265-013-0068-5.
48. Schurch B, de Sèze M, Denys P, et al. Botox Detrusor Hyperreflexia Study Team Botulinum toxin type a is a safe and effective treatment for neurogenic urinary incontinence: results of a single treatment, randomized, placebo controlled 6-month study. J Urol. 2005;174(1): 196–200.
49. Kennelly M, Dmochowski R, Schulte-Baukloh H, Ethans K, Del Popolo G. Efficacy and safety of onabotulinumtoxinA therapy are sustained over 4 years of treatment in patients with neurogenic detrusor overactivity: Final results of a long-term extension study. Neurourol Urodyn. 2015. doi: 10.1002/nau.22934.
50. Rajkumar GN, Small DR, Mustafa AW, Conn G. A prospective study to evaluate the safety, tolerability, efficacy and durability of response of intravesical injection of botulinum toxin type A into detrusor muscle in patients with refractory idiopathic detrusor overactivity. BJU Int. 2005;96(6):848–52.
51. Del Popolo G. Botulinum-A toxin in the treatment of detrusor hyperreflexia. Abstract n 93. ICS annual meeting, Seoul; 2001.
52. Wyndaele JJ, Van Dromme SA. Muscular weakness as side effect of botulinum toxin injection for neurogenic detrusor overactivity. Spinal Cord. 2002;40(11):599–600.
53. Del Popolo G, Filocamo MT, Li Marzi V, et al. Neurogenic detrusor overactivity treated with english botulinum toxin a: 8-year experience of one single centre. Eur Urol. 2008;53(5): 1013–9.
54. Grosse J, Kramer G, Stohrer M. Success of repeat detrusor injections of botulinum a toxin in patients with severe neurogenic detrusor overactivity and incontinence. Eur Urol. 2005;47: 653–9.
55. Gregoriadis G, Ryman BE. Liposomes as carriers of enzymes or drugs: a new approach to the treatment of storage diseases. Biochem J. 1971;124(5):58.
56. Gregoriadis G, Jain S, Papaioannou I, Laing P. Improving the therapeutic efficacy of peptides and proteins: a role for polysialic acids. Int J Pharm. 2005;300(1–2):125–30.
57. Sapra P, Tyagi P, Allen TM. Ligand-targeted liposomes for cancer treatment. Curr Drug Deliv. 2005;2(4):369–81.
58. Gregoriadis G. Engineering liposomes for drug delivery: progress and problems. Trends Biotechnol. 1995;13(12):527–37.
59. Gregoriadis G, Allison AC. Entrapment of proteins in liposomes prevents allergic reactions in pre immunised mice. FEBS Lett. 1974;45(1):71–4.
60. Ebrahim S, Peyman GA, Lee PJ. Applications of liposomes in ophthalmology. Surv Ophthalmol. 2005;50(2):167–82.
61. Kaufman J, Tyagi P, Chancellor MB. Intravesical liposomal (Lp08) instillation protects bladder urothelium from chemical irritation. J Urol. 2009;181, article 539.
62. Tyagi P, Chancellor MB, Li Z, et al. Urodynamic and immunohistochemical evaluation of intravesical capsaicin delivery using thermosensitive hydrogel and liposomes. J Urol. 2004;171(1):483–9.

63. Fraser MO, Chuang Y-C, Tyagi P, et al. Intravesical liposome administration—a novel treatment for hyperactive bladder in the rat. Urology. 2003;61(3):656–63.
64. Tyagi P, Chancellor M, Yoshimura N, Huang L. Activity of different phospholipids in attenuating hyperactivity in bladder irritation. BJU Int. 2008;101(5):627–32.
65. Parkin J, Shea C, Sant GR. Intravesical dimethyl sulfoxide (DMSO) for interstitial cystitis—a practical approach. Urology. 1997;49(5):105–7.
66. Sun Y, Chai TC. Effects of dimethyl sulphoxide and heparin on stretch-activated ATP release by bladder urothelial cells from patients with interstitial cystitis. BJU Int. 2002;90(4):381–5.
67. Bade JJ. A placebo-controlled study of intravesical pentosan- polysulphate for the treatment of interstitial cystitis. Br J Urol. 1997;79(2):168–71.
68. Tyagi P, Hsieh VC, Yoshimura N, Kaufman J, Chancellor MB. Instillation of liposomes vs dimethyl sulphoxide or pentosan polysulphate for reducing bladder hyperactivity. BJU Int. 2009;104(11):1689–92.
69. Chuang Y-C, Lee W-C, Lee W-C, Chiang P-H. Intravesical liposome versus oral pentosan polysulfate for interstitial cystitis/painful bladder syndrome. J Urol. 2009;182(4):1393–400.
70. Chancellor MB, De Groat WC. Intravesical capsaicin and resiniferatoxin therapy: spicing up the ways to treat the overactive bladder. J Urol. 1999;162(1):3–11.
71. Byrne DS, Das A, Sedor J, et al. Effect of intravesical capsaicin and vehicle on bladder integrity in control and spinal cord injured rats. J Urol. 1998;159(3):1074–8.
72. Mandal M, Lee K-D. Listeriolysin O-liposome-mediated cytosolic delivery of macromolecule antigen in vivo: enhancement of antigen-specific cytotoxic T lymphocyte frequency, activity, and tumor protection. Biochim Biophys Acta. 2002;1563(1–2):7–17.
73. Chuang Y-C, Tyagi P, Huang C-C, et al. Urodynamic and immunohistochemical evaluation of intravesical botulinum toxin a delivery using liposomes. J Urol. 2009;182(2):786–92.

Bladder Augmentation: is there an Indication for Mini-invasive Surgical Approach?

14

Giulio Del Popolo and Giovanni Mosiello

14.1 Background

Augmentation cystoplasty (AC) is a surgical procedure that involves the use of bowel segments to increase bladder capacity. AC can be considered as the last option in neurogenic and non-neurogenic bladder dysfunction in those cases where conservative management and minimally invasive treatments have been unsuccessful and exhausted [1, 2]. Neurological patients with neurogenic detrusor overactivity (NDO) should initially undergo medical treatment with antimuscarinics and the addition of intermittent catheterization (IC), usually needed in patients with detrusor-sphincter dyssynergia. If these are unsuccessful, the next step should be intradetrusor injections of botulinum toxin A (BoNT/A) that offer an alternative in those with intractable NDO, even though the effect is only temporary and up to a median period of 9 months. In non-neurological patients, when antimuscarinics fail, BoNT/A, at the lower dosage of 100 U, is indicated, even if there is still a relative risk of urinary retention and consequent catheterization, not always accepted by patients suffering from idiopathic conditions [3, 4]. Alternatively, in non-neurogenic patients with symptoms refractory to other treatments, the neuromodulation may also be attempted [5]; this approach offers a quality-of-life (QoL) improvement comparable with antimuscarinics [6]. Patients who fail treatment with all these modalities are then considered for AC that is the most common indication in neurogenic patients.

G. Del Popolo (✉)
Neurourology Unit, University Careggi Hospital, Florence, Italy
e-mail: delpopolog@aou-careggi.toscana.it

G. Mosiello
Pediatric Urology, Bambino Gesù Hospital, Rome, Italy

© Springer International Publishing Switzerland 2016   187
A. Carbone et al. (eds.), *Functional Urologic Surgery in Neurogenic and Oncologic Diseases*, Urodynamics, Neurourology and Pelvic Floor Dysfunctions, DOI 10.1007/978-3-319-29191-8_14

Generally, AC has been used for the treatment of the low capacity, poorly compliant, or refractory overactive bladder (OAB) [7] and for congenital urological anomalies in pediatric population (i.e., bladder exstrophy). However, in the last decades, the use of AC is decreasing because [7] newer therapeutic approaches are reducing, even if not eliminating, the need for this surgical approach. In the UK, the overall number of AC procedures (ileocystoplasty, colocystoplasty, caecocystoplasty, specified and unspecified enlargement of the bladder) has shown an overall downward trend over the last decade, falling from 192 operations in 2000 to 120 in 2010 [8]. Specifically, the number of ileocystoplasty procedures performed has decreased from 155 in 2000 to 91 in 2010 [8]. In comparison, the number of BoNT/A treatments has significantly increased from around 50 cases in 2000 to 4088 in 2010 [8, 9].

14.2 Indications for AC (Table 14.1)

The main indication for AC is represented by neurogenic and non-neurogenic bladder dysfunction in those cases where conservative management, lifestyle modification, pharmacological therapies, and minimally invasive treatments have failed [1, 2]. The surgical procedure aims to restore urinary storage, protect the upper urinary tract preserving renal function, reduce urinary infection, and provide continence and a convenient method of voluntary and complete emptying in idiopathic patients, while most of neurological patients, particularly patients with spinal cord injury (SCI), need IC [7, 9].

Khastgir et al. found high satisfaction rates and successful surgical outcomes (increase in bladder capacity, reduction in detrusor pressure, and resolution of concurrent reflux) following AC in 32 spinal cord injured patients with refractory neurogenic bladder; Zachoval et al. reported similar outcomes in patients with multiple sclerosis [10, 11].

Kwun-Chung Cheng confirmed the effectiveness of AC in increasing bladder capacity, improving bladder compliance and reducing detrusor overactivity in 40 neurogenic women with 10 years of follow-up. The author emphasizes the preservation of renal function and the low rate of metabolic complications providing a solid evidence of long-term favorable outcomes of this procedure in patients with neurogenic or non-neurogenic bladder dysfunction [12].

Other papers in the literature report satisfactory outcomes of AC (as measured by postoperative symptom scores or urodynamic parameters) in 88% of patients, with a clean intermittent self-catheterization (CIC) rate ranging from 10 to 75% [13–17].

Table 14.1 Neurological and non-neurological patients with possible indications to AC

Neurogenic conditions	Non-neurogenic conditions
Spinal cord injury	Interstitial cystitis
Myelomeningocele	Radiation cystitis
Tethered cord	DO with low-compliance bladder
Multiple sclerosis	Defunctionalized bladder (dialysis)

Another indication for AC includes the management of low capacity and poorly compliant bladder determined by infective diseases (i.e., schistosomiasis, tuberculosis) and inflammatory disorders that may develop after radiotherapy, intravesical or systemic chemotherapy, or interstitial cystitis [13, 14]. Studies on patients suffering from interstitial cystitis/bladder pain syndrome are limited by the small case series and by the variability of results [15–17]. Satisfactory outcomes have been reported in patients with small-capacity bladders caused by Hunner's ulcer disease, with complete pain relief in 63% and improvement in 25%; however, it is well reported that patients may experience pain recurrence also in augmented bladders [15–17]. Although the indication of recent studies in literature seems to be controversial, symptoms related to previous radiotherapy can be treated with AC with a success rate at about 70% [18, 19].

Regarding the treatment of congenital bladder anomalies in pediatric population [20–22], Rubenwolf et al. assessed the long-term results of continent urinary diversion (CUD) and AC in 44 children with irreversible lower urinary tract dysfunction (LUDT) from 1992 to 2007. In this study, an overall complete continence was achieved in 94% of the cohort (95% of patients with CUD and 83% in those with AC), while upper urinary tract and renal function remained stable in 89% and 95%, respectively. Although it is a small study, the results show the effectiveness of AC (and CUD) in children with acceptable long-term complication rates [23].

Another indication for AC is in the setting of renal transplantation, because it is considered better than ileal conduit urinary diversion in terms of protecting the renal allograft from high-pressure reflux nephropathy and consequent graft failure [7, 24, 25]. AC can be performed previously, after or at the time of kidney transplantation because there is no significant difference regarding graft survival between the techniques [26, 27].

As in adults, also in children the main goal of AC is to create a low-pressure catheterizable reservoir. Therefore, surgical indication could be represented by a simple augmentation, aiming to create a continent reservoir, or by a bladder replacement. The choice should be based on:

- Mental and physical status
- Ability to perform self-administered CIC
- Age
- Renal function and its expected evolution during time
- Outlet (bladder neck and urethral) status
- Previous bowel surgery, including appendectomy and ventriculoperitoneal shunt

All these aspects may be more relevant in pediatric patients where a correct choice will allow a long-life improvement.

14.3   Contraindications

Since the procedure involves the digestive tract, the contraindications to AC include intrinsic bowel disease (Crohn's disease, congenital anomalies such as cloacal exstrophy, bladder/bowel tumors, and previous radiotherapy), or conditions resulting in short or abnormal bowel, whereby the removal of a bowel segment will produce further deleterious effects [28]. Another relative contraindication is the reduced manual dexterity or cognitive function leading to an inability to perform CIC. Significant renal impairment is actually a relative and controversial contraindication. In fact, recent studies on children with chronic renal insufficiency and neuropathic bladder submitted to AC showed stable renal function at 1.9-year follow-up in 73 % or its improvement in 18 % (mean GFR 34 ml/min/1.73 m^2) [29].

14.4 Surgical Perspective and Techniques

Among the different surgical techniques, ileocystoplasty is the most used type of bladder augmentation. Mikulicz first described augmentation ileocystoplasty in humans in 1889 [30]. The technique was then popularized by Couvelaire in the 1950s for the management of tuberculous bladders and was further published by Bramble in the 1980s in conjunction with CIC [1]. However, successful use of different segments of bowel, both simple and complex (including cecum, ascending and sigmoid colon, either tubular or detubularized), has been reported (Table 14.2) [7, 31]. Although the bowel segment used can be a matter of preference of the surgeon, the small bowel is the segment of choice due to its ease of handling, obviously if there are no other contraindications. Similar considerations should be applied in patients undergoing redo procedures. In pediatric population, the gastric segments were once popular for augmentation and considered the only possible choice patients with significant renal function impairment or when no other segments were available as in cloacal exstrophy; however, this technique was correlated to higher risk of complications [7, 31–33].

14.5 Preoperative Evaluation and General Principles

History, bladder diary, creatinine, urine analysis, culture, and cytology should be done before surgery. Upper urinary tract should be investigated by ultrasound to identify any anomaly: if hydronephrosis is diagnosed, an upper urinary tract obstruction (i.e., ureteropelvic junction obstruction) should be excluded before AC.

Table 14.2 Advantages and disadvantages of using different bowel segments for AC

Bowel segment	Advantages	Disadvantages
Stomach	Decreases mucus, infection, and stones	Hematuria, dysuria
Ileum	Available	Electrolyte disorders, production of mucus
Ureter	Minimizes mucus, infection, stones, and electrolyte effects	Only in selected cases
Sigmoid colon	Possible use in case other bowel segments are not available	Electrolyte disorders (metabolic acidosis, hypokalemia, low bicarbonate), possible onset of malignancies

Voiding cystourethrography, or better a videourodynamic examination, should be performed to evaluate cystometric capacity, the presence of any diverticula, the function of the bladder neck, and the presence of vesicoureteral reflux, assessing if it develops at low intravesical pressure or during detrusor contraction with high pressure. If videourodynamic is not available, the urodynamic evaluation should be performed in all patients in whom AC is being considered.

Augmentation procedure usually solves the vesico-renal reflux. However, in patients suffering from low-pressure reflux, the problem might persist also after surgery, even if with lower risk of renal damage.

Cystoscopy can be used in selected cases for identifying occult urethral valves, strictures, or unsuspected bladder pathologies, particularly in neurogenic patients.

During the surgical procedure, a minimal amount of bowel should be used. For this reason, detubularization is recommended, as well as a continence mechanism has to be assured in all procedures, open or laparoscopic; finally, in order to avoid stone formation, only readsorbable suture and stapler must be used.

14.5.1 Augmentation Cystoplasty: Open Technique

Classically, AC is performed by an open abdominal approach with coronal or sagittal bivalving of the bladder down to, and anteriorly, the level of the ureteric orifices, with anastomosis of the bowel segment onto the native bladder [1, 7]. In neurological patients all supratrigonal bladder is removed to avoid residual NDO after partial cystectomy and augmentation. The most widely used bowel segment for AC is a detubularized patch of ileum, usually taken about 25–40 cm from the ileocecal valve [1, 32]. If cecum is used, it is often in conjunction with the terminal ileum (ileocecocystoplasty) [33]. In all these techniques, the utilized bowel segment must be opened along the antimesenteric border.

14.5.2 Autoaugmentation and Other Procedures

An alternative to AC is the "so-called" autoaugmentation (detrusor myomectomy) where detrusor muscle is stripped from the bladder mucosa; it is reported that this technique, described for the first time in 1989, achieves an overall success of 50–70 %. It is used mainly in children and a laparoscopic approach may be considered [34, 35]. This technique offers several advantages: short hospital stay, reduced postoperative complications, and no neoplastic risk. Anyway, long-term results are disappointing, and this is the reason why this technique has been widely used by pediatric urologist, where a temporary mini-invasive solution is useful especially in younger children. Another procedure in complicated dysfunction with vesicoureteral reflux is the ureterocystoplasty using a preexisting dilated ureter, but up to 24 % of the patients require revision surgery [36, 37].

14.6   Laparoscopic and Robotic Approach

Modern advances in surgical technique have introduced laparoscopic gastrocysto-plasty and ileocystoplasty [38] and more recently robotic augmentation ileocysto-plasty [39].

Laparoscopic approach was first described by Gill et al. [38] in a series of three patients with small-capacity neurogenic bladders who underwent laparoscopic ileocystoplasty, sigmoidocystoplasty, and cystoplasty with cecum and proximal ascending colon. In this technique, after a Veress needle pneumoperitoneum, a four-port transperitoneal laparoscopic approach is used and an appropriate 15-cm length of bowel is identified. The distal end of the selected bowel segment is marked with an electrocautery. After desufflation, the preselected loop of the bowel is extracted outside the abdomen through a 2-cm extension of the umbilical port incision. Using open technique, the bowel segment with its mesenteric pedicle is isolated, the bowel continuity is restored, and the isolated bowel segment is detubularized along its antimesenteric border. A repair stitch is placed at both the cephalic and caudal end of the bowel patch to facilitate subsequent laparoscopic orientation and the bowel is allocated again into the abdominal cavity. An anteroposterior cystotomy incision is performed using electrosurgical scissors. After suturing the bowel mucosa and mus-cularis with the bladder wall by a full-thickness, single-layer running suture, the blad-der augmentation is completed [38]. A similar surgical approach is used for robot-assisted enterocystoplasty. The robot-assisted laparoscopic technique has well-known advantages (intracorporeal devices with seven degrees of freedom, high-reso-lution, three-dimensional vision) that facilitate intracorporeal dissection and suturing [39]. These minimally invasive procedures are, then, feasible and efficaciously repro-duce the surgical principles of the open enterocystoplasty, minimizing operative mor-bidity, expediting convalescence, and enhancing cosmesis [38, 39]. However, they are associated with increased operative time, even if technological innovation is every day launching on the market more advanced and efficient devices (laparoscopic staplers) which allow a totally intracorporeal bowel isolation and reconfiguration, lowering the impact of manual suturing on the operative time of the whole surgical procedure, thus to render them feasible and easily reproducible. Laparoscopic approaches in pediatric population started in 1999 with comparable operative time respect to open procedure and decreased hospitalization for stoma procedures [40]. A series in 2004 confirmed positive results in 31 patients, including 16 with a history of ventriculoperitoneal shunt [41]. The combination of laparoscopy and open reconstruction gained popular-ity during time, providing improvement in cosmetic outcomes, similar operative time, decreased postoperative stay, and similar long-term outcomes. On the basis of these results, the concerns become philosophical: the combination of laparoscopy and open surgery by Pfannenstiel incision, with a camera through the umbilicus and extracor-poreal reconstruction so avoiding the need for advanced laparoscopic skills, is widely feasible [41]. This induces new significant doubts, especially when the complete intracorporeal surgical technique has to be performed: Is this procedure truly better than others? Is it feasible? Is it safe? Is it effective? [42]. These questions arised inside the group that reported one of the first laparoscopic AC cases in pediatric urology series. The procedure is technically demanding as well as the correct selection approach and postoperative management. Of course the use of robotic approach simplified some technical points in pediatric age too [43]. The operative technique starts always with cystoscopic stent placement, followed by trocar position: open Hasson technique umbilical 12-mm trocar, two 8-mm secondary robotic arm ports laterally, and two assistant ports (12 and 5 mm). In a cohort of six patients of average age of 9.75 years, the mean operative time was 8.4 h, and only one required open conversion [44]. New surgical approaches are available, but it has to be remembered that surgical reconstruction cannot be effective alone to treat bladder dysfunction [45]. However, literature is still lacking of large, prospective, and comparative studies that allow to definitively establish the advantages of mini-invasive AC approaches. In addition, it has to be considered that the expected increase of using BoNT/A injection to treat neurogenic bladder dysfunction will minimize the use of AC in the future years.

14.6.1 Postoperative Follow-Up

After surgery, postoperative management is similar in open or laparoscopic/robotic techniques.

Patient discharge from hospital in neurological patients is from 5 to 7 days after surgery; it depends on general condition and recovery of bowel function. The 24-Ch silicon catheter is removed from 14 to 21 days after surgery: 21 days is preferable. The AC needs some gentle washing with 20 ml of SS to avoid obstruction due to bowel mucous. After removal of the catheter, the AC has a low capacity varying from 200 to 300 ml. However, month after month a progressive improvement of bladder capacity and compliance can be observed. At 6 months, or before, AC reaches a low pressure and a capacity equal or more than 500 ml. We must recommend our patients to avoid overdistension; in fact, some AC ruptures are described, performing regular IC or timed voiding in patients with spontaneous voiding using bladder compression. Videourodynamic and metabolic controls are recommended at 1 year and a scheduled follow-up.

14.7 Complications

Since AC is a major abdominal operation, a variety of early and late complications have been reported in the literature. Early complications include deep vein thrombosis and pulmonary embolism in 7.1 %, small bowel obstruction (3–5.7 %), bleeding requiring reoperation (0–3.2 %), and fistulas (0–20 %). Postoperative myocardial infarction rate is reported in up to 2.7 %, small bowel obstruction of up to 5.7 %, and wound infection of up to 7.1 %.

Finally, mortality rate from AC is reported to be 0–2.7 %, with higher mortality rates in the earlier series and associated with additional procedures [19, 33, 45–47].

Long-term complications include failure of AC, metabolic disturbance, bacteriuria, urinary tract stones, incontinence, intermittent self-catheterization, perforation of the augmented bladder, and carcinoma [10, 20, 21, 48–51].

Failure of AC, which requires a revision surgery, has been reported in 5–42 % of patients [34, 48, 50, 52–59]. Outcomes resulted to be worse in idiopathic detrusor overactivity (IDO), with long-term success in as few as 53–58 % compared with the higher success rates (≈92 %) reported in neuropathic patients [53, 59, 60].

Hyperchloremic acidosis is a dysmetabolic complication, well known by urologists, following urinary diversion; in AC, it is reported with an incidence of 16 % [45, 61]. In case of colocystoplasty, hypokalemia due to secretion of potassium by the colonic patch should be considered [48]. In case of gastrocystoplasty, hypochloremic metabolic alkalosis occurs due to loss of gastric acid in the urine [62, 63]. Nevertheless, with the introduction of the mini-invasive surgical approaches, the use of bowel segment different from distal ileum tract has become obsolete.

AC lowers intravesical pressure and increases bladder compliance during the urine storage phase and, therefore, reflux usually improves or resolves post AC [64].

Moreover, although renal impairment has been considered a significant contraindication, this assessment is now controversial. In neuropathic pediatric patients with chronic renal impairment, undergoing to AC showed no change in renal function at 1.9-year follow-up in 73 % using ileal or colonic segments [29].

A variable number of patients need CIC to achieve a complete emptying of the augmented bladder, and this may vary from 26 to 100 %, with higher rates in the neuropathic patients [33, 45, 56, 65]. CIC can be associated with urinary tract infection (UTI); bacteriuria is reported up to of 75 %, but only 20 % are symptomatic [45]. Daytime and nighttime incontinence may occur following AC. Bed-wetting is attributed to a reduction in urethral closing pressure, relaxation of the pelvic floor muscles, increased nocturnal polyuria urine output, and failure of the sphincter to increase in tone in response to contractions from the bowel patch during sleep, individually or in combination [31, 66, 67]. Large series have published continence rates of 78 % with cystoplasty alone, 85 % with cystoplasty with simultaneous artificial urinary sphincter (AUS), and 90 % with cystoplasty and subsequent AUS [7, 45, 68]. Management of incontinence post AC includes CIC, anticholinergic medications, further reconstructive bladder neck surgery, urinary diversion, or insertion of an artificial urinary sphincter. As reported in literature, these adjuvant treatments ensure a continence rate of 80–100 % [45].

The formation of bladder stones ranges from 3 to 40 % of AC [7, 49] and is secondary to urinary stasis, UTI, and CIC. One study conducted on pediatric patients undergoing AC showed a 15 % rate of bladder calculi [50] which are five times as common in patients who use CIC after AC and ten times as common in patients with Mitrofanoff [51, 69]. Furthermore in cases where AC is combined with ureteric reimplantation, a non-refluxing ureteroneocystostomy should be considered to reduce the risk of upper tract reflux and calculi [51, 69]. Other complications which rarely occur are represented by the formation of diverticula and spontaneous bladder perforation [7, 59].

The latter is a life-threatening complication with a reported mortality of up to 25 % of cases [70]. The most usual site of perforation is the junction between the bowel and bladder wall and rupture may be explained by local ischemia of this area [71]. Most lesions are intra-abdominal, and exploratory laparotomy is warranted in clinical cases of suspected bladder rupture as the diagnosis can often only be made intraoperatively [70, 72].

Cancer risk has been estimated to be 1.2 % with a long latency period (19–22 years) [73–76]. Adenocarcinoma is the most common histologic type although transitional cell carcinomas have been reported too.

Conclusion

AC retains a role in modern urological practice, especially in refractory OAB and in the pediatric population. The long-term outcome complications are well documented in the literature. Although less-invasive procedures such as intravesical injection of BoNT/A are progressively reducing the indication for AC in neurological patients, there is a new trend of patients who are needing long-term solution such as AC, due to a lower efficacy of BoNT/A after several repeated injections so that AC still has a role in the surgical treatment of the low-compliant bladder, and tissue engineering associated with mini-invasive procedure could be the future solution as an alternative to new neuromodulation approaches.

Laparoscopic and robotic approaches to configure AC are feasible, effective, and easily reproducible in high-volume centers where surgical expertise allows a routine adoption of sophisticated techniques requiring bowel management and its reconfiguration.

As a further statement, we should consider that exciting new methods of bladder tissue engineering are under study, and they are likely to play a role in urinary tract reconstruction including bladder augmentation, so that the future is yet to come.

References

1. Bramble FJ. The treatment of adult enuresis and urge incontinence by enterocystoplasty. Br J Urol. 1982;54:693–6.
2. Mundy AR, Stephenson TP. "Clam" ileocystoplasty for the treatment of refractory urge incontinence. Br J Urol. 1985;57:641–6.
3. Popat R, Apostolidis A, Kalsi V, Gonzales G, Fowler CJ, Dasgupta P. A comparison between the response of patients with idiopathic detrusor overactivity and neurogenic detrusor overactivity to the first intradetrusor injection of Botulinum-A toxin. J Urol. 2005;174:984–9.
4. Dmochowski R, Chapple C, Nitti V, et al. Efficacy and safety of onabotulinum toxin A for idiopathic overactive bladder: a double-blind, placebo controlled randomised dose ranging trial. J Urol. 2010;184:2416–22.
5. Vandoninick V, van Balken MR, Finazzi Agro E, et al. Posterior tibial nerve stimulation in the treatment of urge incontinence. Neurourol Urodyn. 2003;22:17–23.
6. Peters KM, Macdiarmid SA, Wooldridge LS, et al. Randomised trial of percutaneous tibial nerve stimulation versus extended release tolterodine: results from the overactive bladder innovative therapy trial. J Urol. 2009;182:1055–61.
7. Biers SM, Venn SN, Greenwell TJ. The past, present and future of augmentation cystoplasty. BJU Int. 2012;109:1280–93.
8. Department of Health, UK. Hospital episode statistics. Department of Health, UK. Available at: http://www.hesonline.nhs.uk. Accessed Aug 2011.

9. Padmanabhan P, Scarpero HM, Milam DF, Dmochowski RR, Penson DF. Five-year cost analysis of intra-detrusor injection of botulinum toxin type A and augmentation cystoplasty for refractory neurogenic detrusor overactivity. World J Urol. 2011;29:51–7.

10. Khastgir J, Hamid R, Arya M, Shah N, Shah PJ. Surgical and patient reported outcomes of 'clam' augmentation ileocystoplasty in spinal cord injured patients. Eur Urol. 2003;43:263–9.

11. Zachoval R, Pitha J, Medova E, Heracek J, Lukes M, Zalesky M, et al. Augmentation cystoplasty in patients with multiple sclerosis. Urol Int. 2003;70:21–6.

12. Kwun-Chung C, Chi-Fai K, Peggy Sau-Kwan C, Chi-Wai M, Bill Tak-Hing W, Lap-Yin H, Wing-Hang A. Augmentation cystoplasty: urodynamic and metabolic outcomes at 10-year follow-up. Int J Urol. 2015. doi:10.1111/iju.12943.

13. De Figueiredo AA, Lucon AM, Srougi M. Bladder augmentation for the treatment of chronic tuberculous cystitis. Clinical and urodynamic evaluation of 25 patients after long term follow-up. Neurourol Urodyn. 2006;25:433–40.

14. Shawket TN, Muhsen J. Treatment of bilharzial-contracted bladder by ileocystoplasty or colocystoplasty. J Urol. 1967;97:285–7.

15. Elzawahri A, Bissada NK, Herchorn S, Aboul-Enein H, Ghoneim M, Bissada MA, et al. Urinary conduit formation using a retubularized bowel from continent urinary diversion or intestinal augmentations: Ii. Does it have a role in patients with interstitial cystitis? J Urol. 2004;171:1559–62.

16. Nurse DE, Parry JR, Mundy AR. Problems in the surgical treatment of interstitial cystitis. Br J Urol. 1991;68:153–4.

17. Van Ophoven A, Oberpenning F, Hertle L. Long-term results of trigone-preserving orthotopic substitution enterocystoplasty for interstitial cystitis. J Urol. 2002;167:603–7.

18. Shirley SW, Mirelman S. Experiences with colocystoplasties, cecocystoplasties and ileocystoplasties in urologic surgery: 40 patients. J Urol. 1978;120:165–8.

19. Smith RB, van Cangh P, Skinner DG, Kaufman JJ, Goodwin WE. Augmentation enterocystoplasty: a critical review. J Urol. 1977;118:35–9.

20. Bhatnagar V, Dave S, Agarwala S, Mitra DK. Augmentation colocystoplasty in bladder exstrophy. Pediatr Surg Int. 2002;18:43–9.

21. Surer I, Ferrer FA, Baker LA, Gearhart JP. Continent urinary diversion and the exstrophy-epispadias complex. J Urol. 2003;169:1102–5.

22. Youssif M, Badawy H, Saad A, Hanno A, Mokhless I. Augmentation ureterocystoplasty in boys with valve bladder syndrome. J Pediatr Urol. 2007;3:433–7.

23. Rubenwolf PC, Beissert A, Gerharz EW, Riedmiller H. 15 years of continent urinary diversion and enterocystoplasty in children and adolescents: the Würzburg experience. BJU Int. 2009;105:698–705. doi:10.1111/j.1464-410x.2009.08908.x.

24. Nguyen DH, Reinberg Y, Gonzalez R, Fryd D, Najarian JS. Outcome of renal transplantation after urinary diversion and enterocystoplasty: a retrospective, controlled study. J Urol. 1990;144:1349–51.

25. Rigamonti W, Capizzi A, Zacchello G, Capizzi V, Zanon GF, Montini G, et al. Kidney transplantation into bladder augmentation or urinary diversion: long-term results. Transplantation. 2005;80:1435–40.

26. Basiri A, Hosseini Moghaddam S, Khoddam R. Augmentation cystoplasty before and after renal transplantation: long-term results. Transplant Proc. 2002;34:2106–8.

27. Dinckan A, Turkyilmaz S, Tekin A, Erdogru T, Kocak H, Mesci A, et al. Simultaneous augmentation ileo-cystoplasty in renal transplantation. Urology. 2007;70:1211–4.

28. Khoury JM, Webster GD. Augmentation cystoplasty. World J Urol. 1990;8:203–4.

29. Ivancic V, DeFoor W, Jackson E, et al. Progression of renal insufficiency in children and adolescents with neuropathic bladder is not accelerated by lower urinary tract reconstruction. J Urol. 2010;184:1768–74.

30. Von Mikulicz J. Zur operation der angebarenen blaben-Spalte. Zentralbl Chir. 1889;20:641–3.

31. Adams MC, Mitchell ME, Rink RC. Gastrocystoplasty: an alternative solution to the problem of urological reconstruction in the severely compromised patient. J Urol. 1988;140:1152–6.

32. Hendren WH, Hendren RB. Bladder augmentation: experience with 129 children and young adults. J Urol. 1990;144:445–53.
33. Whitmore 3rd WF, Gittes RF. Reconstruction of the urinary tract by cecal and ileocecal cystoplasty: review of a 15-year experience. J Urol. 1983;129:494–8.
34. Swami KS, Feneley RC, Hammonds JC, Abrams P. Detrusor myectomy for detrusor overactivity: a minimum 1-year follow-up. Br J Urol. 1998;81:68–72.
35. Cartwright PC, Snow BW. Bladder autoaugmentation: early clinical experience. J Urol. 1989;1(42):505–8.
36. Churchill BM, Aliabadi H, Landau EH, McLorie GA, Steckler RE, McKenna PH, et al. Ureteral bladder augmentation. J Urol. 1993;150:716–20.
37. Johal NS, Hamid R, Aslam Z, Carr B, Cuckow PM, Duffy PG. Ureterocystoplasty: long-term functional results. J Urol. 2008;179:2373–5.
38. Gill IS, Rackley RR, Meraney AM, Marcello PW, Sung GT. Laparoscopic enterocystoplasty. Urology. 2000;55:178–81.
39. Kang IS, Lee JW, Seo IY. Robot-assisted laparoscopic augmentation ileocystoplasty: a case report. Int Neurourol J. 2010;14:61–4.
40. Hedican SP, Schulam PG, Docimo SG. Laparoscopic assisted reconstructive surgery. J Urol. 1999;161(1):267–70.
41. Chung SY, Meldrum K, Docimo SG. Laparoscopic assisted reconstructive surgery, a 7 years experience J. Urology. 2004;171(1):372–5.
42. Lorenzo AJ, Cerveira J, Farhat WA. Pediatric laparoscopic ileal cystoplasty, complete intracorporeal surgical technique. Urology. 2007;69(5):977–81.
43. Gundeti MS, Acharya SS, Zagaya GP. The University of Chicago technique of complete intracorporeal pediatric robotic assisted laparoscopic augmentation ileocystoplasty and Mitrofanoff appendicovesicostomy. BJU Int. 2011;107(6):962–9.
44. Mosiello G, Torino G, De Gennaro M. Laparoscopic Mitrofanoff procedure in children, surgery alone is not effective for the treatment of bladder dysfunction. J Ped Urol. 2015;11(5):301–2.
45. Greenwell TJ, Venn SN, Mundy AR. Augmentation cystoplasty. BJU Int. 2001;88:511–25.
46. Küss R, Bitker M, Camey M, Chatelain C, Lassau JP. Indications and early and late results of intestino-cystoplasty: a review of 185 cases. J Urol. 1970;103:53–63.
47. George VK, Russell GL, Shutt A, Gaches CG, Ashken MH. Clam ileocystoplasty. Br J Urol. 1991;68:487–9.
48. Bandi G, Al-Omar O, McLorie GA. Comparison of traditional enterocystoplasty and seromuscular colocystoplasty lined with urothelium. J Pediatr Urol. 2007;3:484–9.
49. Obermayr F, Szavay P, Schaefer J, Fuchs J. Outcome of augmentation cystoplasty and bladder substitution in a pediatric age group. Eur J Pediatr Surg. 2011;21:116–9.
50. Metcalfe PD, Cain MP, Kaefer M, Gilley DA, Meldrum KK, Misseri R, et al. What is the need for additional bladder surgery after bladder augmentation in childhood? J Urol. 2006;176:1801–5.
51. DeFoor W, Minevich E, Reddy P, Sekhon D, Polsky E, Wacksman J, et al. Bladder calculi after augmentation cystoplasty: risk factors and prevention strategies. J Urol. 2004;172:1964–6.
52. Edlund C, Peeker R, Fall M. Clam ileocystoplasty: successful treatment of severe bladder overactivity. Scand J Urol Nephrol. 2001;35:190–5.
53. Awad SA, Al-Zahrani HM, Gajewski JB, et al. Long-term results and complications of augmentation ileocystoplasty for idiopathic urge incontinence in women. Br J Urol. 1998;81:569–73.
54. Shekarriz B, Upadhyay J, Demirbilek S, et al. Surgical complications of bladder augmentation: comparison between various enterocystoplasties in 133 patients. Urology. 2000;55:123–8.
55. Kockelbergh RC, Tan JB, Bates CP, et al. Clam enterocystoplasty in general urological practice. Br J Urol. 1991;68:38–41.
56. Kreder KJ, Webster GD. Management of the bladder outlet in patients requiring enterocystoplasty. J Urol. 1992;147:38–41.
57. Lewis DK, Morgan JR, Weston PMT, et al. The 'clam': indications and complications. Br J Urol. 1990;6(5):488–91.

58. Kelly JD, Kernohan RM, Keane PF. Symptomatic outcome following clam ileocystoplasty. Eur Urol. 1997;32:30–3.
59. Beier-Holgersen R, Kirkeby LT, Nordling J. Clam ileocystoplasty. Scand J Urol Nephrol. 1994;28:55–8.
60. Hasan ST, Marshall C, Robson WH. Clinical outcome and quality of life following enterocystoplasty for idiopathic detrusor instability and neurogenic bladder dysfunction. Br J Urol. 1995;76:551–7.
61. Koch MO, McDougal WS. The pathophysiology of hyperchloraemic metabolic acidosis after urinary diversion through intestinal segments. Surgery. 1985;98:561–70.
62. Kurzrock EA, Baskin LS, Kogan BA. Gastrocystoplasty: long-term follow up. J Urol. 1998;160:2182–6.
63. Kurzrock EA, Baskin LS, Kogan BA. Gastrocystoplasty: is there a consensus? World J Urol. 1998;16:242–50.
64. Soylet Y, Emir H, Ilce Z, Yesildag E, Buyukunal SN, Danismend N. Quo vadis? Ureteric reimplantation or ignoring reflux during augmentation cystoplasty. BJU Int. 2004;94:379–80.
65. Lockhart JL, Bejany D, Politano VA. Augmentation cystoplasty in the management of neurogenic bladder disease and urinary incontinence. J Urol. 1986;135:969–71.
66. Jakobsen H, Steven K, Stigsby B, et al. Pathogenesis of nocturnal urinary incontinence after ileocaecal bladder replacement: continuous measurement of urethral closure pressure during sleep. Br J Urol. 1987;59:148–52.
67. Akerlund S, Berglund B, Kock NG, et al. Voiding pattern, urinary volume, composition and bacterial contamination in patients with urinary diversion via a continent ileal reservoir. Br J Urol. 1989;63:619–23.
68. Venn SN, Mundy AR. Long-term results of augmentation cystoplasty. Eur Urol. 1998;34 Suppl 1:40–2.
69. Nurse DE, McInerney PD, Thomas PJ, Mundy AR. Stones in enterocystoplasties. Br J Urol. 1996;77:684–7.
70. Couillard DR, Vapnek JM, Rentzepis MJ, Stone AR. Fatal perforation of augmentation cystoplasty in an adult. Urology. 1993;42:585–8.
71. Essig KA, Sheldon CA, Brandt MT, Wacksman J, Silverman DG. Elevated intravesical pressure causes arterial hypoperfusion in canine colocystoplasty: a fluorometric assessment. J Urol. 1991;146:551–3.
72. Sheiner JR, Kaplan GW. Spontaneous bladder rupture following enterocystoplasty. J Urol. 1988;140:1157–8.
73. North AC, Lakshmanan Y. Malignancy associated with the use of intestinal segments in the urinary tract. Urol Oncol. 2007;25:165–7.
74. Soergel TM, Cain MP, Misseri R, Gardner TA, Koch MO, Rink RC. Transitional cell carcinoma of the bladder following augmentation cystoplasty for the neuropathic bladder. J Urol. 2004;172:1649–51.
75. Balachandra B, Swanson PE, Upton MP, Yeh MM. Adenocarcinoma arising in a gastrocystoplasty. J Clin Pathol. 2007;60:85–7.
76. Esquena Fernández S, Abascal JM, Tremps E, Morote J. Gastric cancer in augmentation gastrocystoplasty. Urol Int. 2005;74:368–70.

Index

© Springer International Publishing Switzerland 2016
A. Carbone et al. (eds.), *Functional Urologic Surgery in Neurogenic
and Oncologic Diseases*, Urodynamics, Neurourology and Pelvic
Floor Dysfunctions, DOI 10.1007/978-3-319-29191-8

Printed in the United States
By Bookmasters